FUNDAMENTAL PRINCIPLES
OF CIRCULATION PHYSIOLOGY
FOR PHYSICIANS

FUNDAMENTAL PRINCIPLES OF CIRCULATION PHYSIOLOGY FOR PHYSICIANS

HIROSHI KUIDA, M.D.

Professor of Medicine and Physiology
Chief of Cardiology
University of Utah, College of Medicine
Salt Lake City, Utah

ELSEVIER • NEW YORK
New York • Oxford

Elsevier North Holland, Inc.
Vanderbilt Avenue, New York, New York 10017

Distributors outside the United States and Canada:

Thomonds Books
(A Division of Elsevier/North-Holland Scientific Publishers, Ltd.)
P.O. Box 85
Limerick, Ireland

Library of Congress Cataloging in Publishing Data

Kuida, Hiroshi.
    Fundamental principles of circulation physiology for physicians.

    Bibliography: p.
    Includes index.
    1. Cardiovascular system. 2. Cardiovascular system—Diseases. I. Title.
QP102.K84   612'.1   78-4464
ISBN 0-444-00308-8
ISBN 0-444-00309-6 pbk.

Manufactured in the United States of America

CONTENTS

PREFACE

Cardiovascular diseases produce physiologic derangements that ultimately lead to clinical manifestations. Ideal medical (health) care consists of preventing the disease. Assuming this cannot be or has not been done, optimal medical care consists of sensitive surveillance for clinical clues and specific detection of and intervention in the pathophysiologic processes where feasible, when appropriate, and at the least risk and expense. State-of-the-art medical practice in the second half of the twentieth century has yet to achieve either goal with respect to many diseases.

The aim of this book is to help the reader gain insights into normal physiologic mechanisms of the cardiovascular system and how these are disturbed by various common disease processes with the hope that this will assist the physician achieve more optimal care of his/her patients. It is intended to be a survey useful to general physicians whose concern is broad concepts rather than details. A good friend of mine whom I asked to review this compendium called it a "personal view of cardiovascular physiology" which, of course, it is. The breadth of material covered and the depth of treatment reflects my judgment of the minimum information any physician needs to have to practice cardiovascular medicine on a scientific base. It reflects the 20-year struggle on my part to gain the necessary insights that would permit my helping medical students and physicians at various stages of education/training understand the gross features of cardiovascular physiology. In my attempt to keep complex material simple and comprehensible, I know I have risked inaccuracy. Accordingly, I warn the novice what the sophisticate already knows; that much of what is referred to as knowledge turns out to be something less when examined by better techniques.

HIROSHI KUIDA, M.D.

This book is dedicated to
my deceased sister, Fukiko,
and to my friend, Dr. Murray Rabinowitz,
for their lessons of courage.

1
INTRODUCTION

There, on the sea, is a man nearest to his own making, and in communion with that from which he came, and to which he shall return. For the wise men of very long ago have said, and it is true, that out of the salt water all things came. The sea is the matrix of creation, and we have the memory of it in our blood.

H. BELLOC.
The Cruise of the Nona.
Baltimore: Penguin, 1958.

The cell, the functional unit of life, is a remarkable complex building block. It is estimated that the human body is made up of 100 trillion of them, each of which has the same qualitative requirements for survival and function as an independent unicellular organism, such as the amoeba. The amoeba thrives when environmental conditions are suitable and this is also true for every cell in a complex multicellular organism. Suitable is defined as an environment that has the proper characteristics with respect to temperature, water, oxygen, electrolytes, substrates, and nutrients; a physiologic environment.

In regard to volume, the amoeba lives in a virtually infinite medium, its nearest amoeba neighbor being usually several body diameters away. Thus, there is negligible competition for oxygen and foodstuffs and no problem with removal of wastes, especially carbon dioxide. But the amoeba lives a life of limited options and it is vulnerable to the slightest perturbations of its environment.

The conglomeration of cells and their subsequent evolutionary functional differentiation provided higher organisms far greater flexibility in responding to the vicissitudes of nature, but at the expense of individual cell freedom necessitated by a group response and the requirement for cells to compete for substances in the environment needed for survival. In the beginning, alimentation (assimilation of foodstuffs) and tissue respiration (exchange of O_2 and CO_2) could be accomplished by a common mechanism for enhancing access to substances in the environment by propelling the environment (flow) past cells so that each would be exposed as nearly as possible to the same

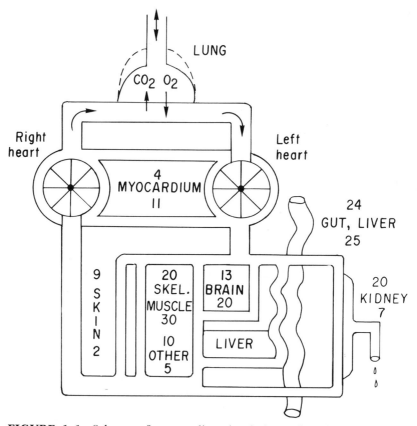

FIGURE 1–1 Schema of mammalian circulation. The wheels represent pumps. The number above each major regional circulatory bed identified is approximate percentage of cardiac output perfusing that bed. The number below is the fraction of total resting body oxygen consumption consumed by that tissue.

concentration of needed materials. Progressive sophistication of organisms led to cells becoming more and more compacted, as well as more and more specialized. The environmental space of each cell became restricted to the point where in higher forms it is only a fraction of the volume of the cell itself. The nutritional substances in such a limited space would be quickly exhausted and the concentration of excretion products rise to toxic levels unless constantly replenished/removed at a rate adequate to maintain normal cell function. It became necessary to provide progressively greater independence of the system for gas exchange from that providing alimenta-

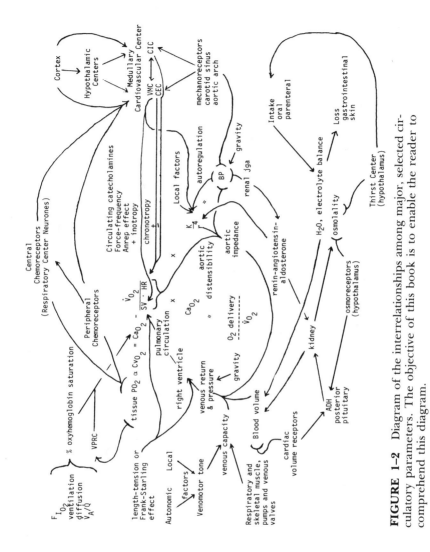

FIGURE 1-2 Diagram of the interrelationships among major, selected circulatory parameters. The objective of this book is to enable the reader to comprehend this diagram.

tion. The circulatory system was open at first, which means that it communicated with the environment and other body cavities and it circulated an undifferentiated fluid that differed little from that of the environment in which it existed. Eventually, however, evolutionary advances led to the system becoming closed. Closure undoubtedly occurred related to the development of more sophisticated circulatory fluids, especially ones containing respiratory pigments, such as hemocyanins and hemoglobin, which markedly enhanced the fluid's oxygen transport capacity. Thus, closure prevented continual loss of these valuable gas-binding substances. Closure meant that the circulation would provide the only means for contact between most of the cells and the external environment, the latter achieved through the development of various interfacing systems. These, in turn, gave nature the flexibility to evolve air breathing and even land dwelling because with the internal environment sealed in, it only remained for the development of interfacing mechanisms with a dry rather than water environment.

Thus, the circulatory system in higher forms shown schematically in Figure 1–1 represents the transport link between the limited watery environment of all the cells of the body and the interfaces with the external environment in the lung (gas exchange, pH regulation), gut (water, nutrition), skin (temperature regulation), and kidney (water, pH balance). Armed with its remarkable gas-binding respiratory pigment, hemoglobin, the function of the circulation is to maintain a physiologic environment for all the cells of the body. This task is accomplished by maintaining an adequate flow of blood through the capillaries in the tissues that maintain favorable gradients for the exchange of the myriad of constituents that are important for cell function between capillary blood and the cell environment. Blood flow, of course, requires an energy source or generator (pump), and getting the blood to and from the various capillary beds requires distribution (arteries) and collecting (veins) systems of tubes.

Lest the simplicity of the anatomic schema in Figure 1–1 be misleading, Figure 1–2 illustrates the complex realities of the multiple interrelationships among the physiologic components of the circulatory system in its most highly developed form. The remainder of the book represents the legend for this figure and its explanation.

2

GENERAL ASPECTS
OF CIRCULATION PHYSIOLOGY

It is therefore necessary to conclude that the blood in the animals is
impelled in a circle, and is in a state of ceaseless movement; that this is
the act or function of the heart, which it performs by means of its
pulse; and that it is the sole and only end of movement and pulse of
the heart.

WILLIAM HARVEY.
exercitatio anatomica de motu cordis et sanguinis in animalibus.
An anatomical dissertation on the movement of the heart and blood in animals.
Frankfurt, 1628.

The function of the circulation is to maintain a physiologic environment for all the cells of the body under all the conditions in which
the body functions. The cellular environment that Claude Bernard
called the milieu intérieur is the interstitial fluid that also is in direct
contact with the capillaries coursing through it. The volume and composition of interstitial fluid reflect a balance between the rate at which
all substances are: (1) delivered to the capillary–interstitial fluid
boundary, (2) either consumed or produced in cellular biochemical
processes, and (3) carried away by the venous or lymphatic systems.
In the case of heat, gain or loss depends on other mechanisms, such
as radiation and convection, as well. The capillary–interstitial fluid
interface represents, therefore, the site where the function of the
circulation is served. The movement of most substances, whether gas,
liquid, or solid, across the capillary endothelial membrane in both
directions depends primarily on diffusion.

DIFFUSION

Diffusion is the phenomenon that results from random thermal motion of molecules. As a consequence of their aimless wandering, molecules collide with one another. Whenever the concentration of a
molecular species is unequal in a given space and no barriers exist,
molecular motion ceases to be truly random. Instead, because of un-

equal collision rates, a net movement takes place that ultimately eventuates in uniform distribution of all molecular species when molecular
motion becomes random again, a state referred to as equilibrium.
Obviously, the net movement is from higher concentration toward
lower and it is this transport that is termed diffusion. In solutions,
both solute and solvent molecules undergo diffusion whenever their
concentrations are not everywhere equal. Diffusion varies directly
with diffusivity or solubility, surface area, and concentration gradient
and inversely with distance as expressed by the Fick equation

$$\frac{dn}{dt} = -DA\frac{dc}{dx}$$

Where dn/dt = Net amount of substance crossing a boundary per
               unit time,
       c = concentration of substance,
      A = cross-sectional area of boundary,
      x = distance,
      D = diffusion coefficent.

The Fick equation states that diffusion transport will be greatest when
surface area is large, concentration gradient high over short distance,
and the substance is highly diffusible. One of the impressive lessons
biology has to offer is the extent to which nature has taken maximum
advantage of these principles in system design. This is particularly
true in terms of achievement of maximum surface area and minimum
distance for diffusion while keeping the cell environment and circulatory fluid volumes small.

While the general principle of diffusion applies to the movement
of substances across the capillary endothelium, we know that the
physicochemical and morphologic characteristics of the capillary endothelium are complex and variable from tissue to tissue and that
deviations from idealized diffusion may occur. For example, water,
ions, and water soluble particles may pass through pores or clefts in
the endothelial membrane whereas lipid soluble substances are able
to pass directly through the substance of the membrane itself. The
renal glomerular capillaries demonstrate impressive fenestration of
endothelium and because of high intracapillary pressure water is filtered through the membrane. In some endothelial cells, other biologic transport processes occur, such as pinocytosis and facilitated
diffusion. In pinocytosis, for example, material is engulfed or im-

bibed on one side of the cell and somehow or other moves across to the other side of the cell where it is discharged.

The surface area for capillary diffusion (A) depends on the number of open (i.e., perfused) capillaries and their geometry (shape, length, radius, etc.). The density (number of capillaries per unit cross section) of perfused capillaries and blood flow direction in neighboring capillaries determine the distance over which diffusion must take place. Because capillary density varies from tissue to tissue, diffusion distance does too. For example, in heart muscle this distance is approximately 7 μ, the diameter of red blood cells, whereas in brain white matter, the distance is several-fold greater. Concentration gradients of all substances depends on the relationship of circulatory transport of each substance to and/or from the capillary bed and cellular consumption or production rate. Transport of a substance to or from the capillary bed in turn is the product of blood concentration of the substance and blood flow.

The unique diffusion coefficient or diffusivity of each substance (D) also plays an important role. For example, approximately the same volume of carbon dioxide is produced by cellular metabolism as is oxygen consumed in a unit of time. The concentration (in the case of gases expressed as partial or percentage of total pressure) gradients necessary for this one-to-one exchange of the two gases are quite different. Carbon dioxide, a highly soluble gas, exits the cell and enters the capillary blood under a pressure difference of only a few millimeters of mercury (mm Hg). For the same volume of O_2 to leave the capillary and get to the cell requires a pressure gradient many times greater.

OXYGEN UTILIZATION AND SUPPLY

Role of Oxygen as a Circulatory Determinant

Of the number and variety of substances carried in blood, the most important to an aerobic organism is oxygen. Indeed, maintenance of adequate tissue oxygen tension can be said to be the prime purpose and function of the circulatory apparatus. When O_2 need is met, all other substances are adequately supplied or removed assuming the environment provides the essential conditions (temperature, water, food) necessary to maintain life. A corollary of the importance of O_2

supply is the elimination of CO_2, the end product of energy metabolism. The oxygen and carbon dioxide levels in arterial blood are determined by the magnitude of effective ventilation (this is called alveolar ventilation, the amount of ventilation that reaches the gas-exchanging pulmonary alveolar–capillary interface). That oxygen level is the more important parameter can be gleaned from: (1) In O_2 deprivation states (e.g., high-altitude dwelling or sojourn) ventilation increases to maintain O_2 levels even though CO_2 level diminishes. (2) Compared to the mammalian situation, fishes markedly hyperventilate. They pass large quantities of water through their relatively inefficient gills to obtain adequate O_2 supply and in the process end up with very low CO_2 levels.

Aerobic metabolism refers to the biochemical processes, shown in Figure 2–1, that are involved in the oxidative combustion of foodstuffs to yield high-energy phosphate compounds (e.g., adenosine triphosphate, ATP) for various biologic processes, heat, and carbon dioxide. The linkage between oxygen utilization and high-energy phosphate compound generation, oxidative phosphorylation, is as fundamental to the animal kingdom as photosynthesis is in plants. The former occurs in the mitochondrion and the latter in the chloroplast.

The earth's modern atmosphere is remarkably uniform in composition with respect to both time and place, providing approximately 21% oxygen, or a partial pressure (P_{O_2}) of 159 mm Hg at sea level and 50 mm Hg at the top of Mt. Everest. In contrast, the P_{O_2} of the seas and other large bodies of water is variable from time to time and place to place. Mammalian mitochondrial P_{O_2} is quite low, on the order of a few mm Hg. Thus, there is a substantial loss of O_2 availability between environment and mitochondria, as is shown in Figure 2–2, mostly accounted for by the large drops between arterial blood (P_{O_2} = 100 mm Hg at sea level) and interstitial fluid (P_{O_2} approximately averaging 20–30 mm Hg) and between the latter and the subcellular organelle. As will be developed in the following section, the adequacy of oxygen availability boils down to the ratio of the level of cellular aerobic metabolism (oxidative phosphorylation) to blood flow.

The oxygen requirements of various tissues differ and vary within a given tissue from one time to another. Intuition alone would suggest the likelihood not only of variable vascularity (i.e., capillary density and number of open vessels) but also of different blood flow rates to

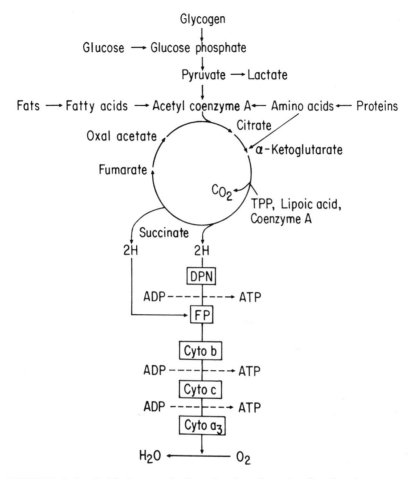

FIGURE 2-1 Oxidative metabolism showing the role of molecular oxygen (at the bottom of the figure) as a proton acceptor permitting oxidative phosphorylation to proceed resulting in the generation of ATP, the biologic energy currency.

tissues, and a mechanism for adjusting each flow rate and/or vascularity to suit particular circumstances of the moment. Perhaps the most vascular and highly perfused tissue in the body is the tiny carotid body. This presumably relates to its chemoreceptor function of sensing the oxygen tension of arterial blood. Other highly perfused and vascular tissues are the kidney and the choroid plexus, tissues in which an ultrafiltrate of plasma is produced in the formation of urine

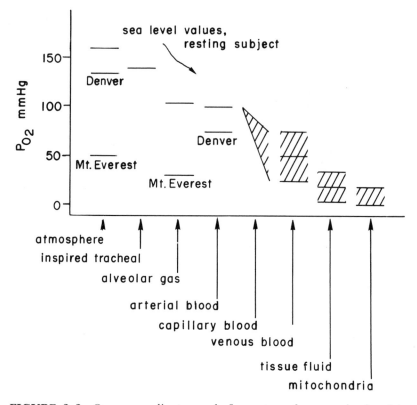

FIGURE 2-2 Oxygen gradient cascade from atmosphere to mitochondria. Cross-hatched areas represent ranges of values, variability depending on specific tissues and on blood flow rate. For example, the lung parenchyma is bathed in a very high P_{O_2}. The compromising effect of altitude dwelling is shown by reduction of P_{O_2} at different levels.

and cerebrospinal fluid, respectively. In these tissues the high flow rates do not relate to a high intrinsic metabolic activity but to their important hemodynamic function. In contrast, contracting heart muscle, while extremely vascular (4000–6000 capillaries/sq mm depending on species), also has a high metabolic activity, thus flow per unit mass is high but flow relative to oxygen consumption is low. At the opposite extreme, fatty tissue predictably has sparse vascularity, low metabolic activity, and low blood flow.

With the exception of tissues where it is determined by other requirements such as those mentioned, blood flow basically is a function of each tissue's inherent oxygen requirement (i.e., its oxidative metabolic activity). The amount of oxygen remaining in the venous effluent from a capillary bed, tissue, organ, or the whole body reflects the extent to which oxygen delivery to that vascular segment exceeds it metabolic requirement. Those tissues with a high venous O_2 content can be said to be highly perfused and those with a low venous O_2 relatively underperfused. The quantity of oxygen in mixed venous blood in the pulmonary artery, accordingly, reflects the state of perfusion of the body as a whole. In normal man at rest, approximately four times more oxygen is transported to the tissues of the body than is consumed in a unit of time. Since only one-fourth the oxygen delivered to the body in arterial blood is utilized, three-fourths returns in venous blood giving rise to a mixed venous oxygen content 75% (P_{O_2} about 50 mm Hg) of what it is in arterial blood.

The physiologic wisdom of what, at first glance, might be thought of as a waste of cardiac energy and blood flow is explicable on the basis of the requirement to maintain physiologic tissue oxygen tension, for the cells of the body exist and carry out their functions in a watery environment, the O_2 tension of which depends on diffusion of O_2 from capillaries.

As stated previously, diffusion of oxygen to cells depends on tension or pressure difference (ΔP_{O_2}), the surface area available, and the distance over which diffusion must occur. However complex and variable from tissue to tissue the microcirculation may be in terms of capillary density, the number of all capillaries being perfused at any given time and how the latter is regulated by the metabolic activity of the tissue, it is clear that there are cells in most tissues that are not exposed to arterial O_2 tension. To the extent that O_2 leaves the blood at the arterial end of the capillary bed there is less at the venous end. In addition, there are differing diffusion distances to consider. Thus, along the course of a given perfused capillary there is a P_{O_2} gradient in the surrounding cylinder of tissue that is highest for cells nearest the capillary at the arterial end and lowest for cells most remote from the capillary at the venous end, the so-called lethal corner. At any given level of tissue metabolic activity, the lower the blood flow rate and the fewer the number of perfused capillaries the greater will be the gradients of oxygen from arterial to venous end and from near the capillary to far from the capillary. These features are illustrated in Figure 2–3. The average tissue oxygen tension will, of course, be some value less than that in arterial blood and probably not much lower than in venous blood. The evidence suggests that venous P_{O2} provides a close estimate of it. Thus, in order that all cells within a tissue are provided with an oxygen tension adequate for normal function, blood flow must be high enough to maintain the oxygen tension of the blood at the venous end of the capillary sufficiently high such that even the cells most distant from the venous end of the capillary will receive an adequate supply.

Oxygen Delivery to Tissues

In 1870 Adolph Fick formulated a simple principle for measuring blood flow that proved to be a powerful tool in physiologic investigations. Fick stated that blood flow could be calculated if the amount of a substance added to or subtracted from the circulation and its concentration in arterial and venous blood are known. Thus, using oxygen as the substance, flow ($\dot{Q}$) can be calculated by the Fick equation as follows

$$\dot{Q} = \frac{\dot{V}_{O_2}}{Ca_{O_2} - Cv_{O_2}}$$

where $\dot{V}_{O_2}$ = oxygen consumption, Ca_{O_2} = arterial blood O_2 content, Cv_{O_2} = venous blood O_2 content.

Some students may find another presentation of this concept easier to understand: Tissues consume oxygen in metabolic processes. Oxygen is transported to tissues by flowing blood. The product of blood flow rate ($\dot{Q}$) and the oxygen concentration of arterial blood (Ca_{O_2}) represents the amount of oxygen delivered to the tissue in a unit of time

$$\text{Delivery} = \dot{Q} \cdot Ca_{O_2}.$$

Of this total amount of oxygen delivered, some is consumed by the tissue ($\dot{V}_{O_2}$) and the balance (surplus) is carried away in venous blood. The sum of these two, whatever the partition, must be equal to the aforementioned amount of O_2 delivered. In steady state, the effluent (venous) blood flow rate, whatever its oxygen concentration, must be the same as the arterial inflow rate; thus

$$\dot{Q} \cdot Ca_{O_2} = \dot{V}_{O_2} + \dot{Q} \cdot Cv_{O_2}.$$

Rearranging

$$\dot{V}_{O_2} = \dot{Q} \cdot Ca_{O_2} - \dot{Q} \cdot Cv_{O_2}$$

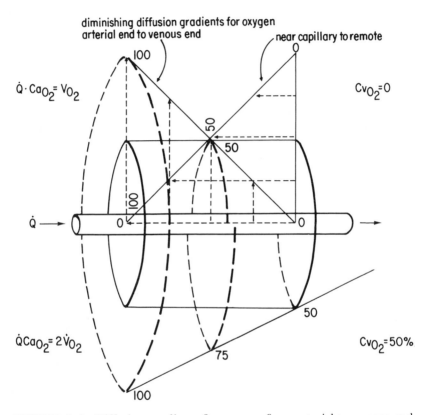

FIGURE 2-3 Diffusion gradients for oxygen from arterial to venous end and from near capillary to remote surrounding a capillary through which flow ($\dot{Q}$) proceeds from left to right. A cylinder of tissue surrounding the capillary is shown. The radius of this cylinder is variable in different tissues and is determined by the distance between adjacent capillaries. In the upper half of the cylinder a situation is depicted where the oxygen delivery to the capillary, the product of blood flow and arterial O_2 content ($\dot{Q} \cdot Ca_{O_2}$), is equal to oxygen consumed in the cylinder ($\dot{V}_{O_2}$). The short half-cone shows the rapid decline of O_2 availability ending in a venous content of zero. The shape of the cone is not intended to be quantitatively accurate. In the lower half, O_2 delivery is twice consumption due to doubling of blood flow (Ca_{O_2} remaining constant). In this situation the oxygen gradient (cone) is more gradual for both arterial–venous and near–remote (not shown). Venous O_2 level, therefore, is still 50% of arterial that allows for much higher average tissue P_{O_2}.

and since it is $\dot{Q}$ we wish to know

$$\dot{Q} = \frac{\dot{V}_{O_2}}{Ca_{O_2} - Cv_{O_2}}$$

the famous Fick equation for calculating blood flow rate.

We can substitute cardiac output (CO) for $\dot{Q}$ in the previous equation to calculate the blood flow to (or from) the whole body, but since the amount of O_2 in each of the myriad of venous tributaries may be different, we have to know what the average value is for all of them. A sample of such value is referred to as mixed venous blood ($C_{\bar{v}}$) and optimally is obtained from the pulmonary artery where all venous effluents converge after being mixed in the right ventricle.

The Fick equation can be rearranged to provide better insight into the determinants of the oxygen content of venous effluent blood. The latter is important because it represents the closest estimate of average tissue oxygen tension

$$Cv_{O_2} = Ca_{O_2} - \frac{\dot{V}_{O_2}}{\dot{Q}}.$$

By assuming that venous blood O_2 content is linearly related to venous blood P_{O_2} (a fair assumption) and that the latter is a close estimate of tissue P_{O_2}, we can substitute tissue P_{O_2} for Cv_{O_2}:

$$\text{Tissue } P_{O_2} \, \alpha \, Ca_{O_2} - \frac{\dot{V}_{O_2}}{\dot{Q}}.$$

Thus, at any particular arterial blood O_2 content, tissue P_{O_2} is determined by the ratio of O_2 consumption to blood flow. This is true for any capillary, tissue, organ, and for the whole body.

The equation also makes it clear that in tissues with variable O_2 consumption, unless flow increases in direct proportion to increasing O_2 consumption, tissue P_{O_2} will fall. Skeletal and cardiac muscle exhibit the widest range of O_2 requirement and therefore fluctuations in flow. Another important factor in the adjustment of blood flow to metabolic need is the regulation of the number of capillaries that are perfused at any moment. Such adjustment keeps diffusion distances from capillary to cells appropriate to O_2 demand. The other term in the equation describing the determinants of tissue P_{O_2} is the arterial blood O_2 content. The determinants of this physiologic variable will be discussed in the next section, but it is predictable that whenever this is diminished (such as by anemia or hypoxemia, reduced oxygen in blood, Chapter 14) tissue P_{O_2} will fall unless there is a compensatory increase in cardiac output or a reduction in $\dot{V}_{O_2}$. Such increases in flow indeed do occur when ambient O_2 tension or oxyhemoglobin concentration fall, such as with high-altitude exposure, anemia, or lung disease. Chronic hypoxemia itself is a potent stimulus for increased red cell production to counteract this effect. There is even evidence suggesting that compensatory effects such as decreases in O_2 consumption and shifts in the oxyhemoglobin dissociation curve may occur when oxygen availability or delivery is compromised.

Role of Hemoglobin in Oxygen Transport

The most dramatic way to emphasize the importance of hemoglobin is to point out that in its absence, oxygen would be carried dissolved in plasma and just to supply the oxygen consumption of a sleeping human being (about 250 ml/min) would necessitate a cardiac output (Chapter 7) of approximately 80 liters/min. To deliver the same amount of O_2 that is normally delivered in blood in a resting human (about 1000 ml/min) would require an output of over 300 liters/min! Thus, the evolution of hemoglobin was no less important to mobility and to land dwelling than of lung, heart, and autonomic nerves.

Oxygen is a relatively poorly soluble gas that comprises about 21% of the atmosphere. According to the gas law, it therefore exerts a partial pressure at sea level of $0.21 \times 760 = 159$ mm Hg, or of the total barometric pressure of the atmosphere at sea level, 760 mm Hg, oxygen accounts for $159/760 = 21\%$. The amount of gas that will dissolve in water (or plasma) is a function of its partial pressure and solubility constant, which for O_2 is 0.023 cc/ml/atmosphere. Thus, at sea-level oxygen partial pressure of 159 mm Hg, only 4 ml of O_2 $(0.023 \times 159/760 \times 1000)$ would be present in each liter of water (plasma) allowed to come to equilibrium. For reasons that will not be covered here, the partial pressure of O_2 at the gas exchanging alveolar–capillary interface in the lung is reduced from 159 to 104 mm Hg. This results in only 3 ml of O_2 that can be carried in solution in each liter of plasma devoid of red cells and explains why an output of over 80 liters/min would be required to transport 250 ml of O_2/min.

The hemoglobin in red blood cells combines reversibly with O_2 in a most remarkable way. When hemoglobin combines with all the O_2

it can (this is referred to as full or 100% saturation), each gram carries 1.34 ml of O_2. In the blood of normal man residing at sea level, each 100 ml of blood (slightly less than half red blood cells) contains about 15 gr of hemoglobin. This means that instead of 3 ml O_2/liter of blood, $15 \times 1.34 \times 10 = 201$ ml O_2 is carried by hemoglobin, making a total of $201 + 3 = 204$ ml O_2/liter of blood. Thus, hemoglobin exaggerates the oxygen carrying capacity of the blood of normal man at sea level by some 70-fold! This is why with a modest cardiac output of some 6 liters/min, far more O_2 is delivered to the body, $6 \times 204 = 1224$ ml O_2/min, than is consumed at rest.

There are other characteristics of hemoglobin that need to be mentioned although their detailed treatment usually falls within the purview of respiration physiology. The ability of hemoglobin to bind oxygen reversibly instead of being a linear function of oxygen partial pressure (P_{O_2}) is sigmoid. This S-shaped relationship, illustrated in Figure 2–4, has great biologic significance. It means that at higher (above 70 mm Hg) O_2 partial pressure, binding is strong; whereas at lower (below 50 mm Hg) P_{O_2}, it is weak. This characteristic favors O_2 uptake in the lung capillaries where P_{O_2} is high and O_2 release in tissue capillaries where P_{O_2} drops suddenly, due to the outward diffusion gradient. Other factors in the systemic and pulmonary capillary beds contribute to enhance this property. For example, increased carbon dioxide partial pressure (P_{CO_2}), acidity, and higher temperature, conditions present in tissue capillaries, all enhance O_2 release whereas the opposite effects, which are present in pulmonary capillaries, augment O_2 binding. Thus, the function of hemoglobin as an oxygen carrier is multiplied to maximal efficiency in what basically are two opposite tasks, loading and unloading!

The wisdom commonly ascribed to Mother Nature really has more to do with the effect of time and accidents. There has been life on earth for a few billion years. The average sojourn of a species on earth is reckoned to be about a million years, long enough for a great deal of natural selection, adaptation, and many accidental mutations. For example, there is a species of fish that habitates lightless underwater caves that has lost its eyes. The llama, a dweller of the South American altiplano (10,000–20,000 ft) has hemoglobin the dissociation curve of which is significantly left-shifted; that is, its ability to bind O_2 is maintained at the lower P_{O_2} of high altitude.

We now know that there is a substance in red cells, 2,3-DPG (2,3-

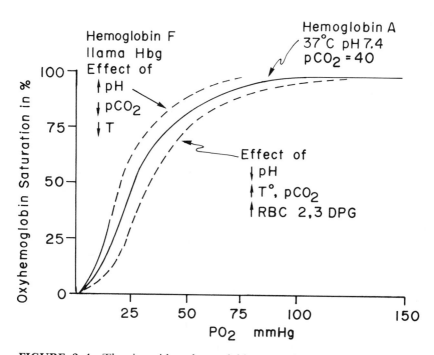

FIGURE 2–4 The sigmoid oxyhemoglobin saturation curve (solid line) for adult (A) hemoglobin. Saturation is the ratio of O_2 content of blood at any P_{O_2} to which it is exposed to that blood sample's maximum capacity to bind O_2 (blood O_2 capacity). Other hemoglobins (F, llama) have different binding characteristics compared to hemoglobin A (under the same controlled conditions) and changing conditions as indicated by arrows also alters the curve (dotted lines) of hemoglobin A.

diphosphoglycerate) that has the effect of shifting the sigmoid curve to the right which, of course, aids in O_2 unloading in the tissues. In other words, this substance has the same effect as increased CO_2, $[H^+]$, and temperature. The important thing is that in a variety of clinical circumstances where O_2 transport is compromised, such as anemia, heart failure, chronic hypoxemia, etc., 2,3-DPG levels in red blood cells have been found to be elevated.

Another feature of hemoglobin is the fact that its dissociation characteristics are different in the fetus (hemoglobin F) compared with that in adults (hemoglobin A). Obviously, the fetus obtains its oxygen from the placenta. Not so obvious is the fact that the fetus lives in a chronic state of potential relative (to the adult situation) hypoxemia (Chapter 14). The placenta is a marvelous exchange device but it lacks the efficiency of lungs in gas exchange, especially of oxygen. From the Fick diffusion equation, the factors involved in placental gas transfer include: surface area, oxygen partial pressure difference between maternal and umbilical arterial blood, the distance separating them in the chorionic villi, and gas solubilities. There is one other factor not accounted for by diffusion, the chemical characteristics of hemoglobin F.

The oxyhemoglobin dissociation curve of fetal blood is left-shifted compared to that of adults, similar to the situation in the llama. One reason for this is that fetal red cells contain less 2,3-DPG. This shift facilitates the placental transfer of oxygen from maternal to fetal blood because at any P_{O_2} fetal red cells have a greater affinity for O_2 than do maternal. This consideration becomes very important for fetuses of pregnancies occurring under conditions of low P_{O_2}, such as residency at high-terrestrial elevations or disease conditions (chronic lung disease or congenital heart disease with venoarterial shunting) associated with arterial hypoxemia.

The left-shifted dissociation curve, while it represents an advantage for the fetus as far as acquisition of oxygen in the placenta is concerned, presents a problem as far as oxygen unloading in the tissues is concerned. Recalling the equation describing the determinants of average tissue P_{O_2}

$$\text{Tissue PO}_2 \; \alpha \; \text{CaO}_2 - \frac{V_{O_2}}{CO}$$

what means are available to enhance O_2 delivery in the face of the unloading problem should be apparent. Oxygen content of arterial blood (Ca_{O_2}) can be enhanced at any partial pressure by increasing the concentration of red blood cells (a condition referred to as polycythemia) and, therefore, of hemoglobin. This is exactly what occurs in the fetus. One of the first things that happens in the newborn is that the extra red cells of the relative polycythemic state are eliminated after birth when air breathing increases P_{O_2}. Rapid destruction of surplus red cells is what produces so-called physiologic jaundice (hyperbilirubinemia) of the newborn.

There is another way to obviate fetal hypoxemia. The ratio of V_{O_2} to cardiac output will be minimal when the former is low and the latter high. It is now known that fetal oxygen consumption per gram of body weight is reduced and cardiac output increased relative to the adult situation. Thus, threatened fetal hypoxemia is avoided by nature's manipulation of each component in the previous equation in such ways that the fetus is provided an adequate supply of oxygen.

Yet another remarkable aspect of the evolution of oxygen transport is the discovery that the oxyhemoglobin dissociation curves of various animal species varies as a function of body size. In the range of body mass encompassed by the elephant at the one extreme and the shrew at the other, there is progressive rightward shift of the dissociation curves under the same conditions of temperature, pH, and P_{CO_2}. This adaptation means that smaller species have enhanced oxygen availability at the tissue level (albeit at some, presumably minor, disadvantage with regard to O_2 uptake in the lungs). The teleologic sense of such an arrangement is that enhanced unloading of oxygen associated with a right-shifted curve represents a valuable mechanism for satisfying the higher (as much as sixteen-fold) oxygen consumption of tissues characteristic of smaller species.

CERTAIN PHYSICAL ASPECTS OF FLOW AND FLOWING BLOOD

Flow, Velocity, and Cross-sectional Area Relationships

In a closed circulatory system under steady-state conditions, the flow rate at each cross section carrying the total flow is everywhere equal. The cross-sectional area of the system in man varies from a minimum of 3–4 sq cm at the aortic and pulmonary valves to perhaps 2000 sq cm at the level of the systemic capillaries. Velocity of flow at a given flow rate is inversely proportional to area

$$\text{Velocity} = \frac{\text{flow rate}}{\text{Area}}$$

That is at a given flow, the product of velocity and area is a constant; if one goes up, the other must go down proportionally. Because flow is discontinuous emerging from the ventricles, average systolic flow velocity in the aortic root and main pulmonary artery is approximately 100 cm/sec during ejection. In the capillaries, flow is reasonably steady at about 0.5–1.0 mm/sec in the systemic and 1.0–1.5 mm/sec in pulmonary capillaries. Assuming capillaries to be approximately 1 mm in length, the time available for gas exchange between red cells and tissue fluid is about 1–2 sec. Burton made the astonishing calculation that it takes 1⅔ yr for 1 ml of blood to pass through a single systemic capillary! Because there are approximately several billion systemic capillaries and perhaps one or two billion pulmonary capillaries that the cardiac output (5–6 liters) is able to pass through the capillary bed cross section in 1 min. Assuming there are 3 billion capillaries, the flow in each would amount to approximately 3×10^{-8} ml/sec. The exchange of gases can easily be accomplished in less than 1 sec in both capillary beds because of the huge surface involved (estimated 70 sq m in the lung capillaries) and short diffusion distances. Despite the large surface areas for diffusion capillaries provide, the volume of blood required to fill capillaries is surprisingly (and beneficially) small; less than 100 ml in the lungs and 500 ml in the body at rest or 10% of the total circulating blood volume.

Blood Flow Patterns

Liquids and gases have in common flow patterns that differ depending on a number of factors. Energy input (force) required to produce flow of a gas or liquid is minimal in so-called laminar flow. In laminar flow, gas or fluid molecules move in a smooth, orderly array wherein infinitely thin layers have an ordered velocity relationship in space or across the cross section of the tube, as shown in Figure 2–5. Velocity is zero at the tube wall. There is an infinitely thin layer of molecules in contact with the tube wall that flows not at all. Velocity of adjacent laminae progressively increases toward the tube axis where velocity is greatest and quantitatively is twice the average velocity of all laminae. The velocity profile of all concentric laminae from tube wall to center is parabolic in shape.

FIGURE 2–5 Laminar flow in a tube showing just a few of a large number of infinitely thin concentric flow laminae moving from left to right, each at a different velocity ranging from zero at the tube wall to maximum at the tube axis. The average velocity is half the maximum and the profile of laminar velocities across the tube from wall to axis is parabolic.

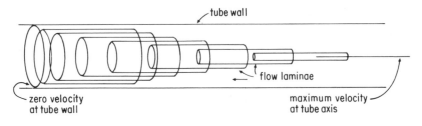

tube wall

flow laminae

zero velocity
at tube wall

maximum velocity
at tube axis

When certain conditions are met, laminar flow breaks down and becomes turbulent. As the term implies, there is no order in this type of flow and all molecules tend to flow at more or less the same velocity. Thus, the velocity profile becomes squared off. There is a great deal of random mixing and eddy formation across the cross section quite unlike molecules in a given laminar flow sleeve that tend to stay put in that position, mixing only by diffusion. More energy is required to produce turbulent flow compared to laminar, or frictional energy loss in turbulent flow is much greater. Such energy losses may appear in the form of sound (Chapter 5), which may reach very high levels (e.g., jet aircraft takeoff).

Sir Osborne Reynolds studied the factors that influence whether flow will be laminar or turbulent and determined the following relationship:

$$Vc = \frac{R\eta}{\rho r}.$$

The critical velocity (Vc) at which flow changes from laminar to turbulent is determined by the ratio of Reynolds number (R) and fluid viscosity (η) to density (ρ) and the tube radius (r). At Reynolds' numbers in excess of 1000 (mean, not maximal velocity), flow is usually turbulent.

Reynolds' numbers have been calculated for different vascular sites and these are usually less than 1000 under normal resting conditions. However, critical velocity may be exceeded in the aortic root or pulmonary artery under conditions of increased cardiac output. In such situations, systolic ejection may produce an audible murmur. Turbulence also occurs just downstream from localized points of obstruction or narrowing in tubes. Such turbulence is also localized and results from the formation of eddys at the point where the stream of higher velocity issuing from the narrowed portion rapidly decelerates as the radius increases. This type of turbulence occurs at velocities less than critical and is the mechanism for sound produced by an aeolian harp. Obstructive lesions in the cardiovascular system commonly produce murmurs and pulmonary airway obstructions produce wheezes.

Viscosity of Blood

Blood is a complex circulatory fluid because of plasma proteins and the suspension of formed elements (red and white blood cells and platelets). These alter the behavior of flowing blood in a variable manner depending on their concentration, the velocity of blood flow and the bore of blood vessels. These variables affect the viscosity· of blood. Viscosity has to do with the slipperiness (or, more precisely, the lack of it) of a liquid; it is defined as the ratio of shear stress to shear rate. In other words, how much force is required to overcome the frictional resistance within a liquid to produce a constant level of velocity difference between one layer of fluid and adjacent ones (i.e., velocity gradient)?

Solving the Poiseuille equation (Chapter 8) for viscosity yields

$$\eta = \frac{\Delta P \pi r^4}{\dot{Q} 8L} \; .$$

In rigid capillary tubes (radius, r, and length, L, are constant) with laminar flow, viscosity coefficient (η) is the ratio of driving pressure (ΔP) to flow ($\dot{Q}$). A Newtonian fluid is one that obeys this law of viscosity, its coefficient of viscosity is constant at a given temperature. The law applies to most homogeneous fluids. Blood plasma or serum qualify as Newtonian fluids and have a viscosity, relative to that of water, of approximately 1.8.

Whole blood exhibits a number of unusual (the term anomalous is commonly used) viscous properties that render it non-Newtonian. At normal red blood cell concentration (approximately 40–50% by volume), whole blood relative viscosity is approximately 3–4. Viscosity increases with increasing red blood cell concentration and also with the presence of high concentrations of large protein molecules called macroglobulins. There are disease conditions wherein red blood cell concentration may reach 80% or more. In vitro (glass viscometer) viscosity at such levels maybe elevated threefold (i.e., tenfold that of water).

Fortunately, there is another feature of blood flowing in blood vessels that ameliorates the effect of red blood cells on viscosity. This feature is called the Fahraeus–Lindqvist effect. What these investigators observed was that the relative viscosity of blood was constant in tubes greater than 0.3 mm diameter, but in progressively smaller tubes viscosity diminished as a function of tube bore approaching that of plasma. Whittaker and Winton subsequently observed that the apparent viscosity of blood of varying red cell concentrations between 20 and 80% was less when measured in a dog hind limb preparation, as compared with that obtained in a glass viscometer. Furthermore,

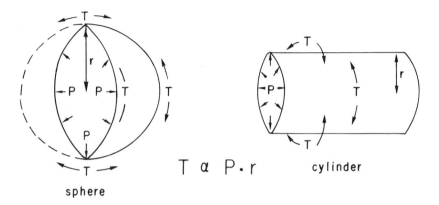

T α P·r   sphere   cylinder

FIGURE 2–6 Law of Laplace and cardiovascular structures. Pressure, force per unit area (P), inside a tube or cavity is balanced by tension, force per unit length (T), in the wall that varies directly proportional to radius of curvature (r). In heart chambers during contraction wall tension rises actively creating fluid pressure. In elastic vessels, the fluid pressure created by heart contraction produces passive vessel wall tension proportional to radius and in muscular vessels the same passive tension is enhanced by an active tension component that tends to diminish tube bore at any given luminal pressure.

the higher the red-cell concentration, the greater was the discrepancy. Thus, it seems that when blood flows in very small tubes, the viscosity is less than what one would be led to expect, obviously a situation that favors flow with the least energy expenditure. The mechanism of this effect is thought to be related to the axial streaming of red cells in small tubes. By traveling faster than plasma in small vessels, red cells occupy a smaller volume (i.e., the concentration of red cells in blood flowing in small vessels is lowered) thus minimizing the effect of red-cell suspension on viscosity.

Tension in the Walls of Blood Vessels

Anyone who has blown up a toy balloon or inflated a tire or sports ball of some type recognizes there is some relationship between inflation pressure and the tenseness of the chamber wall. The physical principle involved was formulated by Laplace in 1821 and is shown in Figure 2–6.

$$T = P \cdot r \text{ (for a cylinder)}$$

Where T = wall tension, dynes/cm, P = pressure, dynes/ sq cm, r = radius of curvature, cm.

The equation states what one could easily observe, that at any given internal pressure, wall tension is a function of radius. This explains why the tip of a partially inflated elongated toy balloon feels soft compared to the wall of the fully inflated section, despite a common internal pressure throughout. It also explains why overinflation eventuates in rupture or bursting (such as of a soap bubble). That is to say, as either or both P and r increase, T rises to the point where the structural competence limit of the material is exceeded and blowout occurs.

This principle has much relevance to the cardiovascular system. It should be obvious that the wall tension in the aorta of the giraffe (high P and large r) must be many orders-of-magnitude greater than in a hummingbird. Capillaries are able to withstand high pressure (up to arterial level) without bursting (at least usually) because of their microscopic size. Diseases that diminish the structural integrity of the aortic wall lead to aneurysm formation (fusiform or sac-like dilatation). This creates the ingredients of a vicious circle of escalating wall tension and diminishing wall strength as r increases, culminating in rupture. Veins in the legs during dependency, especially when valves are incompetent, are subjected to high intraluminal pressure; this combined with dilatation leads to high vein wall tension. The latter weakens vein wall and further dilatation occurs creating the ingredients of a vicious cycle of escalating wall tension leading to varicose veins and chronic venous insufficiency.

3
CARDIAC ELECTRICAL ACTIVITY

Our search for a well-differentiated system of fibers within the sinus, which might serve as a basis for the inception of the cardiac rhythm, has led us to attach importance to this peculiar musculature surrounding the artery at the sino-auricular junction (Fig. 6, A, 2). In the human heart the fibers are striated, fusiform, with well-marked elongated nuclei, plexiform in arrangement and imbedded in densely packed connective tissue—in fact, of closely similar structure to the *Knoten* (AV node, described by Tawara in 1906 and confirmed by authors) . . . we feel justified in expressing the opinion that it is in them that the dominating rhythm of the heart normally begins.

ARTHUR KEITH AND MARTIN FLACK.
Journal of Anatomy and Physiology, 1907.

Muscle is a biologic engine. An engine is a device that has the ability to convert energy in one of various forms to a form capable of performing work. The energy transduction that muscle accomplishes is the conversion of chemical energy to mechanical (with heat generated as a by-product). This transduction requires an intermediate triggering step involving electric excitation of the muscle cell membrane. This triggering process might be thought of as being analogous to the electrically induced spark necessary to ignite the fuel–air mixture of internal combustion engines. The big difference in the muscle engine is that excitation of the muscle membrane does not lead to a combustion process that liberates energy. Indeed, the cellular combustion process, oxidative phosphorylation, is going on all the time in mitochondria generating high-energy adenosine triphosphate, ATP. Depolarization of the muscle membrane initiates a chemical mechanism, calcium release, that allows ATP to participate in the isothermal chemomechanical process of contraction. Quite clearly, both processes, the electric and mechanic, and their linkage are important in consideration of muscle physiology. While most of what is known about the electrophysiology of muscle derives from work done in nerve and skeletal muscle, the amount of information obtained from specific studies in cardiac and smooth muscle is rapidly increasing.

Muscle cells share with nerve cells the property of excitability, the ability to propagate an electrical impulse along its length. A biologic electric impulse is called an action potential, and the development of knowledge concerning the physiology of action potentials represents a brilliant chapter in the annals of physiologic science and technology.

The secret to the phenomenon of excitability is locked in the cell membrane. Just what it is about the membranes of excitable cells that confers this property is not known with finality, but there is no doubt that it relates to mechanisms responsible for maintaining particular distributions of ions on the inside of the cells, as compared with the extracellular fluid, and how the forces that maintain those distributions can undergo dramatic change to produce, as well as to propagate, an action potential.

The intracellular ionic composition of all cells in the body differs markedly from that of the interstitial fluid in which they are bathed. This is particularly true of the reciprocal transmembrane distribution of sodium (Na^+) and potassium (K^+) ions, the former being high on the ouside while, conversely, potassium is high on the inside. Apparently there are compelling reasons to invoke an energy-consuming metabolic Na^+–K^+ ionic pump in the membrane to explain these distributions because they exist against their passive diffusion and electric potential gradients. It has been found that most cells, irrespective of excitability, have a transmembrane electric potential with the inside being negative with respect to the outside. This potential is largely owing to the permeability of the membrane to K^+, which produces what is termed the potassium equilibrium potential, E_K. Thus, even if unequal transmembrane distribution of ions account for the presence of a resting membrane potential, unequal distribution by itself cannot explain the property of excitability. Otherwise, liver cells, renal tubular cells, and even red blood cells would be excitable too.

An action potential is characterized by the sudden explosive localized alteration of the membrane voltage that exists in a polarized but quiescent or resting cell when it is depolarized to a certain threshold level by an electric or mechanic stimulus. During an action potential, the inside at a sharply localized locus transiently becomes positive. This sudden localized reversal of membrane polarity (depolarization) reflects an increase in membrane permeability to sodium ion that permits an influx of this ionic species (sodium inward current). Thus, depolarization is dominated by the sodium equilibrium potential, E_{Na}, which is positive. This effect is believed to be due to abrupt opening (activation) of gates in sodium ion conducting channels. The gates to these sodium channels apparently begin closing again almost as fast as they are opened (this is called inactivation) and potassium channels begin opening because an efflux of K^+ ensues that in nerve and skeletal muscle causes the membrane to quickly revert to its resting state of internal negativity. The action potential moves along the membrane because the presence of an action potential at any particular locus of the membrane depolarizes the membrane surrounding that locus to threshold potential, advancing the action potential in all directions. This advancing mechanism is referred to as electrotonic spread. The mechanism by which depolarization to threshold causes the gates of sodium channels to be explosively opened and the latter causes potassium channels to open is not known. There is, thus, a domino effect where the electric energy for spreading the phenomenon derives from the phenomenon itself (i.e., it is self-propagating) analogous to the spread of fire where the heat of the flame brings adjacent objects to kindling temperature.

Nerve and skeletal muscle cell action potentials are characterized by repolarization being almost as quick as depolarization. Cardiac muscle action potentials are quite different in that while depolarization is abrupt (although not quite so rapid as in nerve and skeletal muscle), repolarization is remarkably delayed and it occurs slowly (Figure 3–1). Instead of a few milliseconds, cardiac cells, depending on heart rate, may have action potentials lasting a few to several hundreds of milliseconds! The phenomenon is accounted for by a plateau (so-called phase 2) in the action potential following the initial depolarizing spike (phase 0) and rapid, initial, incomplete recovery (phase 1). The mechanism for this plateau is thought to result primarily from calcium ion (Ca^{++}) inward current.

The prolonged cardiac action potential has great physiologic significance. One characteristic common to nerve and skeletal and cardiac muscle is the fact that an action potential cannot be superimposed on a preexisting one, or, once the cell is depolarized, it cannot be reactivated until it returns to the polarized state (phase 3). As with shooting an arrow, the bow string has to be pulled back before each firing. The interesting paradox raised by this analogy is that no one would consider the pulled bow string the resting condition. Thus, during an action potential the cell is said to be refractory to a second

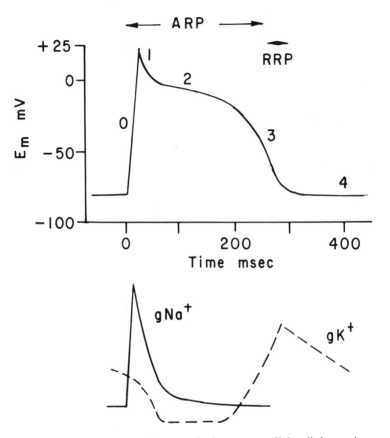

FIGURE 3–1 A representative ventricular myocardial cellular action potential. The phases are descriptively termed: upstroke (0), overshoot (1), plateau (2), repolarization (3) and resting (4). These refer to the membrane voltage (Em) changes that occur during the action potential presumably based on the approximate changes in membrane conductances (g) for sodium and potassium shown below (not shown for other ions). A depolarized cell (phases 0, 1, 2, and about half of 3) is refractory to a subsequent depolarizing current of any strength. This period is referred to as the absolute refractory period (ARP). During the latter part of phase 3 the cell can be depolarized again if a stronger-than-threshold stimulus is applied, a period termed the relative refractory period (RRP).

depolarizing stimulus. The long duration of cardiac action potentials confers an equally long refractory period. Thus, unlike the situation in nerve and skeletal muscle where stimulus frequencies up to 50–100/sec are possible, cardiac muscle is markedly limited as far as the frequency of repetitive stimuli to which it will respond. Cardiac action potential duration automatically shortens as heart rate increases, but even in the smallest mammals, such as the shrew and mouse, heart rates of 400/min (7/sec) are relatively (compared to nerve action potential frequency) slow. The tiniest hummingbirds, however, may have heart rates up to 1000/min (17/sec).

The duration of the contractile process in cardiac muscle is directly related to and, in fact, is about the same as the duration of the action potential (Figure 3–2). This, combined with the syncytial nature of the cardiac mass (see the following) as far as electric activation is concerned (once begun, an action potential will depolarize the entire cardiac mass assuming it isn't extinguished in the atrioventricular [AV] node), means that there can only be a one-to-one relationship between electric excitation and contraction. Thus, cardiac muscle cannot be tetanized the way skeletal muscle can (Chapter 5); that is, repetitive action potentials cannot be delivered to the heart to produce a summated mechanical contraction. The advantage of this arrangement for a pump that has to operate incessantly, making upwards of four billion strokes during a lifetime, should be obvious. The heart beats automatically in an organized and coordinated way essentially as a motor unit, it has periods of rest and recovery automatically alternating with each contraction, and it has built-in safeguards against unduly rapid rates.

In the nervous system, the action potential represents the quantum or unit of communication, messages depending on which ones and the number of individual cells activated and the frequency of action potentials within each cell. In muscle, including heart muscle, the membrane action potential represents the electric disturbance that sets into motion the biochemic processes that lead to the mechanic process of contraction of the contractile machinery. Quite obviously, there is a mechanism for getting an action potential to each and every cardiac cell in a repetitive and coordinated manner.

ORIGIN AND SPREAD OF CARDIAC EXCITATION

The heart beat results from a wave of electric current spreading over the heart, which in mammals originates in a collection of specialized cardiac cells located high in the right atrium at the junction of the superior vena cava called the sinoatrial (SA) node. The ability of SA node cells to initiate an electric impulse spontaneously is appropriately termed automaticity. Thus, the SA node is the normal pacemaker of the heart. The source of electric current that initiates SA node cell discharge is due to an electrophysiologic phenomenon that is variously called slow diastolic depolarization, pacemaker potential, or phase 4 depolarization. It refers to a spontaneous gradual discharge (depolarization) of these cells from the maximum resting potential achieved during the process of cell membrane repolarization, as shown in Figure 3–3. The ionic basis for this depolarizing current has to do with the changing permeability characteristics of the SA node cell membrane to sodium and/or potassium. When one cell undergoes this process to the point of threshold whence it suddenly depolarizes completely, a self-propagating wave ensues that travels from cell to cell across electric bridges, variously called tight junctions, gap junctions, or nexuses, which are characterized by low electric resistance. Thus, from the electric point of view, the anatomically individual cells of the whole heart function as though a continuum and the term functional syncytium is used to describe this characteristic.

As the self-propagating depolarizing current spreads from cell to cell in exponentially increasing numbers, a moving boundary of electric potential difference is established, the interface of which is the voltage difference between cells already depolarized and those still in the polarized or resting state yet to be excited. This wave front of electric activation spreads over the atria in a more-or-less smooth, radial manner in about 50–100 msec. Sometime, but probably early,

FIGURE 3–2 Top: Cardiac muscle cellular action potentials. Dotted lines show effect of increasing frequency (i.e., heart rate) shortening action potential duration automatically. Center: Tension development in cardiac muscle, cell or sarcomere associated with depolarization. Note relative slowness in peak tension development and duration tied to depolarization. Dotted lines show effect of shortened action potential duration associated with higher frequency reducing peak tension development. A. Control conditions. B. Effect of changing conditions (experimental interventions such as adding Ca^{++} or adrenalin to preparation producing positive inotropy) under the same conditions of muscle length and stimulus frequency. Note increased rate of tension development resulting in higher peak tension. Below: Curves of developed tension (as from above) at different muscle lengths, the length-tension effect, solid curve A under control conditions. Dotted curve B: Increased peak tension at any length resulting from positive inotropy as from B above. Dotted curve C: Decreased tension resulting from intervention, such as depriving preparation of adequate oxygenation (not shown above), a negative inotropic effect. The solid and dotted arrows show that in all three curves there is a length-dependent and length-independent mechanism for altering tension.

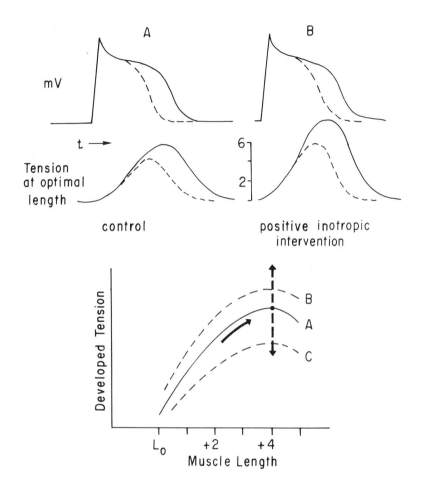

during this interval, the impulse, possibly traveling via specialized internodal tracts, arrives at the AV node. The AV node is a small specialized cardiac structure situated low in the atrium near the ostium of the coronary sinus. Ordinarily, the AV node and bundle of His (so-called junctional tissue) represent the only electric connection between the atria and the ventricles. Therefore, they form the solitary conduction pathway over which the depolarizing current must pass in order that ventricular excitation can follow atrial. These structures and their approximate anatomical location are illustrated in Figure 3–4. (Clinical conditions do exist, however, where accessory, either nodal or nonnodal A-V pathways do exist and function. Birds have a specialized conduction ring around the AV valves that facilitates AV conduction.)

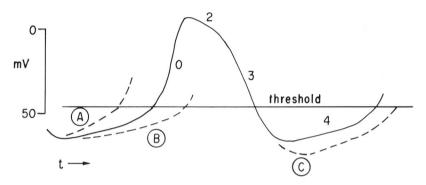

FIGURE 3–3 Cellular action potential in SA node (only one cell need undergo this for successful excitation of the heart but all cells in the SA node have this potential). Striking feature is spontaneous, progressive, slow depolarization during phase 4. This is termed the pacemaker potential because when threshold potential is reached as a consequence of it a regenerative action potential occurs that depolarizes neighboring cells by electrotonic spread. The heart rate (frequency of repetition of SA node action potentials) obviously would be determined by the rate or slope of phase 4 depolarization as in A or B (faster and slower rate, respectively), the magnitude of maximum (negativity) of resting membrane potential as in C and by the threshold level.

Contraction (tension development) of atrial cardiac muscle is a slow process (> 200 msec) compared to the brief inteval (< 100 msec) during which all atrial cells receive electric activation (i.e., are depolarized). The atrial muscle mass, therefore, is able to contract nearly as a unit before the onset of ventricular contraction because while

FIGURE 3–4 Diagrammatic sketch of cardiac electric conduction system with (left) and without (right) cardiac anatomical landmarks. SVC, IVC, RA, LA, RV, LV—self-explanatory; CS—coronary sinus; IAS—interatrial septum; SAN—sinoatrial node; AVN—atrioventricular node; His B.,—His bundle; RBB, LBB, right-and-left bundle branches.

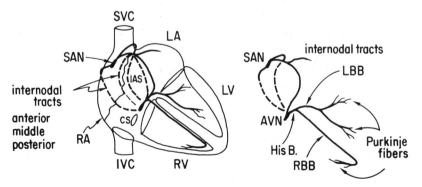

atrial contraction is occurring the AV node and the specialized conducting system (see the following) delay transmission of the depolarizing impulse to the ventricles allowing atrial contraction to be completed. The retardation of impulse transmission through the AV node results from slow condition velocity associated with the small diameter of its fibers and the reduced magnitude of resting membrane potential that lowers action potential upstroke rate and propagation velocity. These intrinsic mechanisms are modulated by physiologic factors, particularly the degree of vagal tone (Chapter 12). Strong vagal stimulation can completely block impulse transmission through the AV junction; contrarily, abrogation of vagal tone (such as by the drug, atropine) permits a high rate of impuse traffic through junctional tissue.

Specialized Conduction System and Ventricular Activation

There are perhaps as many as six to seven times more cells in the ventricular mass as compared with atrial. If electric activation of the ventricles were to occur only on the basis of cell-to-cell spread in the same manner as of atria, the process might require as much as nearly 1 sec, despite the somewhat more rapid conduction velocity in ventricular fibers. This would have dire consequences, and would seriously limit effective cardiac function in larger animals. This emphasizes the value and physiologic function of the specialized conduction system, especially in animals with large hearts. For example, this system permits the ventricles of an elephant heart weighing 20 kg to be activated in 150 msec, less than double that of a human heart weighing a mere 0.3 kg! (Hearts of the largest whales can weigh as much as tenfold the body weight of a man!)

The specialized conduction system of the ventricles consists of the His bundle, the left and right bundle branches and their major arborizations, and the extension peripheral Purkinje net. This system consists of large, high-conduction-velocity fibers that provide rapid, as well as widespread, dissemination of the depolarizing wave, and that permit ventricular depolarization in man to be completed in about the same interval as atrial (60–90 msec) despite the much larger mass of muscle. Because Purkinje fibers are distributed on the endocardial surfaces, as well as within the walls of both ventricles, the general direction of spread of activation is from inside to out, but the geometry of distribution otherwise is sufficiently complex and there are enough intra- and interspecies variations in other details of the sequence and direction of spread that it is impossible to generalize. For example, in humans the overall direction of ventricular activation is from base toward apex, but in bovines it is just the opposite. As the atria, electric depolarization of all ventricular cells occurs so rapidly (< 100 msec) compared to the long duration of mechanical systole (200–400 msec) that the ventricular myocardium contracts essentially as a unit.

When 6–7 billion individual cells are depolarized during a 60- to 80-msec interval by a spreading boundary of activation disseminated by a widely arborizing conduction system, preferentially to one surface of asymmetrical hollow structures of such complex geometry as the ventricles, a great deal of electric activity is going on in different parts of the heart and in all directions simultaneously. Careful measurements have been made of activation sequence in several species utilizing multiple closely-spaced electrodes that confirm the complex nature of the spread of excitation. However, there does seem to be some stereotyped order in normal activation within each species. Gross alterations in sequence are possible without serious alteration of ventricular function because Purkinje fibers spread the impulse reasonably rapidly (90–150 msec) and widely, no matter where the impulse orginates. This is why a cardiac rhythm of ventricular origin is consistent with reasonably normal function, and explains why it is possible to pace the heart artificially through electrodes contacting the ventricular myocardium irrespective of location.

Ventricular Repolarization

While it is conceptually accurate to describe the multiple, complex, simultaneous moving activation boundaries as waves or fronts in the sense that the process both overall and in its component parts proceeds in some identifiable chronologic sequence and direction, this is not the case with repolarization. The sudden depolarization of the cell membrane during activation depends on each cell being depolarized to threshold by a neighboring cell. There is no such requirement for transmission of repolarization. Once depolarized, each cell is more or less independent of all other cells with regard to the time course over which it returns to the resting state. As with all biologic phenomena, there is variability in action potential duration among ventricular cells. Since this may be so for neighboring, as well as for far separated, cells, it is quite clear that there is no obligatory order or sequence for the repolarization process for the ventricles as a whole or any of their parts. Thus, electric recovery of the ventricular mass is not the synchronized wave-like process that activation is, and it is less amenable to sequence analysis. It is not to say each cell is not subject to a number and variety of factors that may have an effect on action potential duration; nevertheless, it is hardly surprising that the overall process of the electric recovery of the ventricles is distributed over a much longer time interval (250–400 msec) compared to that required for activation.

4
ELECTROCARDIOGRAPHY

I have sought a method in which, as far as possible, the construction of a new curve could be avoided, and finally, to offer an instrument which primarily would satisfy the requirements of inscribing the electrocardiograms of human beings in approximately, at least, its correct proportions.

This instrument—the string galvanometer—is essentially composed of a thin silver-coated quartz filament, which is stretched like a string, in a strong magnetic field. When an electric current is conducted through this quartz filament, the filament reveals a movement which can be observed and photographed by means of considerable magnification.

WILLEM EINTHOVEN.
Pflügers Arch. Physiol., 1903.

The clinical application of hemodynamic concepts and techniques followed by some decades their basic development. With respect to the electric activity of the heart, in contrast, clinic application actually preceded basic physiologic knowledge and developments in the field. This resulted from the development of the string galvanometer by Willem Einthoven at the turn of the century. This recording instrument was sensitive enough without electric amplification to detect minute voltage changes resulting from the electric activity of the heart using electrodes placed on the extremities. That such electric activity existed and could be recorded in man had been determined previously by Augustus Waller in 1887 with a mercury capillary electrometer. Einthoven's instrument was a major factor in the growth of knowledge of cardiac electric activity.

Einthoven's original records showed that during each heart cycle, five distinct waves or deflections could be recorded from the body surface. He designated these deflections with letters from the latter part of the alphabet: P for the first, T for the last and QRS for the major, complex, triple deflection in between. The correct significance of these waves was soon recognized as representing: P, atrial activations; QRS, ventricular activation; and T, ventricular recovery or repolarization. The understanding of the cellular physiologic basis of electrocardiography lagged behind, awaiting the development of new techniques; but as an empiric diagnositic tool, the electrocardiogram (ECG) proved to have great clinical utility. While the physiologic basis for electrocardiography is now reasonably well established (although still incomplete), the empiric or so-called pattern recognition approach became deeply ingrained in clinical medicine because of its unequivocal practical value.

MECHANISM OF BODY SURFACE RECORD

There are two basic reasons why it is possible to record electric signals of the heart beat from the body surface: (1) the asymmetry of the geometric–chronologic aspects of the wave of excitation spreading over the heart and of the repolarization process that produce changes in the electric field of the body, and (2) the property of the body as a volume conductor. The latter refers to the simple fact that the various tissues of the body provide a conducting medium owing to the presence of ions (electrolytes) in watery solution. Electric events occurring in a volume conductor produce electric field changes that are transmitted (conducted) to the body surface. Thus, no matter where or how electric currents are generated in the body, the electric field changes they produce will be detectable from the body surface, assuming currents are of sufficient strength or suitable amplification and resolution are provided by recording instrumentation. To be sure, the body is not a perfectly homogenous volume conductor (the lung is quite a bit less conductive than blood, for instance), but this is a complication, not a deterrent. Also, the skin offers high resistance to current transmission from body to recording electrodes but this too can be overcome with suitable coupling (impedance matching) techniques.

If the heart were a hollow sphere of uniform thickness activated uniformly from the entire endocardial surface instantaneously and it lay in a homogenous conduction medium, little or no electric activity reflecting the excitation process would be recorded from electrodes placed on remote sites on the body surface! This is a significant, if hypothetical, observation because it provides important insight into the factors that contribute to events of cardiac electric activity actually being recordable from the body surface. When a depolarizing wave traverses the same thickness of the same mass of muscle at the same speed in exactly (180°) opposite directions, the events are not reflected at distant bipolar electrodes because the electric forces generated (alterations in electric field) cancel each other. Because in the previous hypothetical spherical situation this applies to every opposed pair, it is understandable why the entire process produces negligible, if any, voltage differences between two remote electrodes, no matter where they are placed.

Thus, one thing we can say about the real heart in the real body is that recordable electrocardiographic deflections reflect either voltage differences (recordable as current flow) between surface electrodes that are due to uncancelled electric forces (to the extent cancellation occurs) associated with the origin and spread of the electric process and recovery therefrom, inhomogeneities in volume conduction or both. The fact and extent of cancellation is not widely appreciated. The rapid and widespread dissemination of activation by the Purkinje network initially to the inside surface of hollow chambers (ventricles) means that the potential for cancellation exists, and it has been estimated that as much as 70% of the activation of the ventricular myocardium may be unexpressed on the body surface! This means that what is recorded of ventricular activation is only the residue of what are actually more extensive self-cancelling electric forces. The asymmetry of both the anatomy of the heart and of the pattern of dissemination (activation sequence) of the depolarizing wave of excitation by the Purkinje system account for most of noncancelled forces appearing at the surface.

ELECTROCARDIOGRAPHIC DEFLECTIONS OR WAVES

Cancellation notwithstanding, the electrocardiogram does reflect overall electric activation and recovery therefrom in a way that the average effect of the total population of individual depolarizations is preserved. As a matter of fact, one way to think about electrocardiographic deflections is that they represent a time-dependent frequency distribution of voltage differences among total populations of cells, only a sample of which (uncancelled forces) is recorded. An analysis taking this simple-minded approach is shown in Figure 4–1 and explained in the following text.

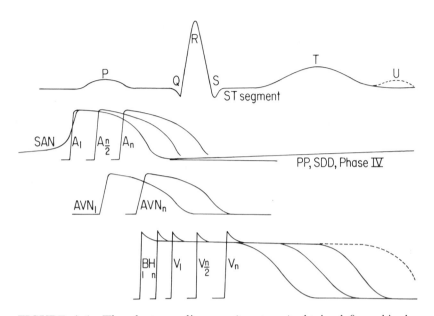

FIGURE 4-1 The electrocardiogram (top trace) obtained from bipolar electrodes on the body surface—say on opposite sides of the chest—reflects the time varying voltage between the electrodes during a single heart cycle. It can be thought of as an electric statistical record of the magnitude of voltage difference among cells, each of which can only be in one of two states: on (polarized) or off (depolarized) as reflected in the cellular action potential. Only a few selected ones of these are shown below from the sinoatrial node (SAN), atrioventricular node (AVN), bundle of His (BH), and ventricle (V). 1 = first cell activated of that tissue, $n/2$ = midpoint activated cell, n = final activated cell. Note ECG deflections relate to progressive increase then decline of voltage differences among populations of cells. See text for amount of cancellation of such differences resulting in no surface deflection—such as atrial repolarization. Note also: mass of His bundle and AV node are too small to be reflected on surface records, slow conduction through very minute mass of AV node and nnite delay between BH and ventricular activation due to bundle branch and Purkinje system conduction. P, QRS, T, and U represent ECG deflection nomenclature. The U wave is thought to reflect Purkinji system repolarization reflecting their long action potential duration.

The P Wave

When all cardiac cells are in the electrically resting or polarized state, obviously there is no potential difference among them; hence there is no deflection (so-called isoelectric baseline). The origin in the SA node and earliest phases of atrial activation represent insufficient tissue mass to produce a surface deflection, but as an exponentially increasing number of atrial cells are depolarized by the rapidly spreading wave, a voltage difference among atrial cells appears and rises to a maximum when half of those for which there is surface expression are depolarized and the remainder are still at resting potential. Since spread is rapid relative to the long duration that cells remain depolarized, as more than half the cells are activated, the deflection on the surface recedes again towards zero from the peak because when all cells are depolarized by the spreading wave, there is again no longer any difference among them despite the fact that they are at a different (i.e., depolarized) electric level. Thus, what is seen on the ECG of atrial activation is a small, gradually rising and falling deflection lasting 60–100 msec. Atrial repolarization, on the other hand, is rarely seen on surface records. The explanation usually given for this is that it is buried in the more obvious QRS complex, which follows atrial activation. While this is undoubtedly true, it cannot be the only explanation because repolarization is also absent when the QRS wave is separated from the P wave by delaying AV node conduction beyond normal or blocking it completely (such as by vagal stimulation). This must mean that the repolarization process is so distributed or self-cancelling compared to activation that the voltage differences among the repolarizing cells lack sufficient magnitude to cause a systematically identifiable ECG deflection.

The QRS Complex

Intuition alone should lead you to suspect that ventricular activation, cancellation notwithstanding, would produce a far greater electrocardiographic disturbance than of atrial, and this is usually the case. However, the difference is not what you might predict based on the difference in mass of tissues involved. (This should have been the first clue of cancellation effects, others of which include: (1) the appearance of large amplitude P waves with right atrial enlargement even though the mass of atrial tissue is still far less than of ventricular, (2) the absence of change in QRS amplitude in autopsy-proven cases of significant ventricular hypertrophy, and (3) discrepancies between the magnitude of electric forces comparing activation and recovery.)

The QRS complex (it is called this whether or not all individual component waves are present) of the electrocardiogram denotes the period during which the depolarizing waves spreading from the His bundle activate the entire ventricular myocardium. It starts and usually ends at the isoelectric baseline, but exceptions are common. Particular patterns of QRS deflections in the various leads (see the following) are commonly used to infer gross characteristics of activation sequence. There is no electrophysiologic rationale for this; rather, it is based on correlation of particular patterns with specific experimental observations or with autopsy-proven pathologic processes. Prolongation of the period of ventricular excitation takes the form of a widened QRS complex (> 100 msec) and is indicative of delay in transmission of the depolarizing wave somewhere below the level of the bifurcation of the His bundle. A block in the His bundle itself could not be distinguished from AV node block without special techniques. Block of either of the two main bundle branches produces characteristic stereotyped alterations in QRS and T wave forms, but this is not the case with conduction disturbances in the periphery that produce variable QRS changes without obligatory alteration of T waves.

As in the case of atrial activation, peak QRS deflection (preferably of an orthogonal lead) reflects the instant when roughly half the ventricular mass is depolarized (by whatever complex routes), for as more and more fibers reach this state the surface deflection returns toward its neutral (isoelectric) position, indicating regression of potential difference among the cells as they reach the depolarized state. This is the so-called J point or the beginning of what is called the ST segment.

The ST Segment

Usually the ST segment is characterized by electric silence (no deflection) between the J point and the beginning of the T deflection. This is because all ventricular cells are and remain at the plateau (phase 2) potential for a relatively long duration before repolarization commences even in the earliest-activated fibers. It is common, however, to find exceptions to this in perfectly normal people. Thus, the notion that ST deflections of one kind or another reflect indicators of specific cardiac disease is tenuous. It is generally true that seriously injured cells develop leaky membranes and either are unable to sustain depolarization (phase 2 or plateau) the way ventricular fibers normally do or their resting potential is diminshed. If significant numbers of them either have a different resting potential or begin to return towards resting potential immediately following depolarization, an ST deflection is bound to occur. Whether such ST deflections are positive or negative seem to have to do with which of these mechanisms obtains or whether the injured cells are predominantly endocardial (ST depression) or epicardial (ST elevation) in location.

The T Wave

The process of electric recovery or repolarization takes much longer than depolarization, both in individual cells and for the ventricles as a whole. The surface record of this process, the T wave, is normally a gradually rising and falling wave of some duration reminiscent of a normal frequency distribution curve. The peak T deflection must reflect that instant when there is maximum uncancelled voltage differences among the cells owing to half the cells of the electrically manifest ventricular mass having returned to resting potential while the remainder is still depolarized. As more and more cells repolarize, the T deflection recedes progressively. This process does not depend on cell-to-cell sequence but probably neither is it totally random. The fact that the voltage–time product (area) of the T wave commonly exceeds that of the QRS deflection suggests that there is less cancellation of repolarization compared with depolarization forces. There is no doubt that the whole process of recovery is much more vulnerable to the number and variety of perturbations, for there is a wide spectrum of unrelated conditions that produce alterations in the magnitude, direction, and time course of the T wave. It is not at all uncommon to see records where one is hard put to identify any T deflection at all similar to the situation with atrial depolarization. This certainly does not mean that the ventricular mass is not undergoing repolarization, it is only that body surface expression of it is self-cancelling. At the other extreme are records that show T waves of giant proportions even though activation is normal. This must mean that there is less than the usual amount of cancellation that allows so much voltage difference to be expressed. A similar mechanism (lack of cancellation) applies to the large amplitude–long duration QRS complexes resulting from abnormal activation sequence associated with beats originating in a ventricular ectopic focus or from block of the main bundle branches.

CARDIAC ELECTRICAL VECTORS

When one visualizes a perfectly spherical object, the direction of one's perspective makes no difference—a round object looks the same from any direction. This is not the case with asymmetric objects, which are infinitely variable in appearance, depending on the angle from which they are viewed. The complex moving boundaries of cardiac excitation do not represent an object in a literal sense; but, when all the multiple independent forces at each instant are averaged, the uncancelled process has spatial, as well as chronologic, components that during each cycle inscribe an asymmetric time–space loop. The latter is what has shape. Obviously, as an asymmetric spatial process, it will appear different depending on the angle from which it is viewed. The loop of a single cycle has some average value in terms of voltage magnitude and direction; it is a vector quantity and there is one for the P, QRS, and T waves. These vectors appear different depending on the three planes (dimensions) from which they can be recorded. Vectorcardiography is the branch of electrocardiography that has as its concern the time–space loops themselves, instantaneous vectors during the cardiac cycle, or the averaged vectors. An average vector can be represented by an arrow (it has a tail and head end) of length proportional to magnitude of the vectoral force and pointed in the appropriate direction in space. This arrow for each of the three main complexes (P, QRS, and T) will cast a shadow on a plane, however oriented, if a light were shone from behind the arrow toward the plane perpendicular to the orientation of the plane. The significance of this is that electrocardiographic body surface leads are equivalent to such planes in the sense that they see by the magnitude and direction (polarity) of deflections the electric analog of such shadows.

ELECTROCARDIOGRAPHIC LEADS

While the electric activity of the heart can be recorded from placement of a pair of electrodes (bipolar record) almost anywhere on the body (except both on one extremity), one of the first things Einthoven discovered was that electrocardiographic deflections differed depending on the placement and polarity of electrodes, and he realized the chaos that would result from lack of standarization and uniformity in recording. Accordingly, he established at the outset arbitrary conventions for recording the three bipolar limb leads. These, the Einthoven triangle leads, became standard, and their use continues to the present. Nine additional leads were added later based largely on the work of Frank Wilson in the mid-1930s. The additional leads improve the diagnostic resolution of the technique; and these also have been universally adopted. Unlike bipolar leads, where the difference in voltage between two leads is recorded, Wilson introduced what are called unipolar leads wherein one electrode, the so-called central terminal of Wilson, is at or near null or zero potential by combining inputs from several extremity leads, voltage differences among which tend to cancel each other out. This near-zero potential is compared against the voltage changes of the other so-called exploring electrode that is placed either on an extremity (unipolar limb leads) or on the chest wall (precordial leads).

Another arbitrary convention that Einthoven established for standard leads was the polarity of bipolar leads. Einthoven apparently liked to see positive QRS deflections, because the polarity he chose results in positive deflections in all three standard leads in the majority of normal people. In the so-called Einthoven triangle electrode arrangement, as shown in Figure 4–2, lead I compares the voltage between the two upper extremities with the left arm positive. In both lead II, right arm versus left leg, and lead III, left arm versus left leg, the left leg is positive. It is assumed that these leads provide an equilateral triangulation of cardiac electrical activity in the frontal plane with lead I being perpendicular to the long axis of the body. Addition of the three unipolar limb leads, V_R, V_L, V_F, provide six views of electric activity in the frontal plane in 30° increments (Figure 4–3). The unipolar precordial leads are placed on specific anatomic sites on the anterior to left lateral chest wall to provide six horizontal plane views in 15° increments from anterior to left lateral.

Why 12 leads, 3 leads, or any other number are used? There are serious research efforts currently underway directed at determining whether there is something worth the cost and trouble involved to be gained from large number, multiple electrode array recording (as many as 192 leads in one case!). This approach is called body surface mapping. It is too early to tell what the ultimate applicability of this approach might be. Clearly, there is nothing magic about the number

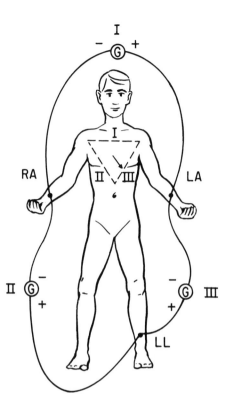

FIGURE 4–2 Electric hookup for recording Einthoven—now called standard—frontal plane ECG leads. G refers to recording instrument's galvanometer. The so-called Einthoven equilateral triangle is shown on the anterior chest wall indicating the relationship of the orientation of the three leads. The arrow represents a typical normal mean QRS vector that would be reflected in predominantly positive QRS deflection in all three leads but least in lead III since the arrow is nearly perpendicular to that lead, angled only slightly towards the positive pole.

of leads. Only one lead is sufficient for rhythm analysis and minimum of three perpendicularly oriented leads to determine the spatial (three-dimensional) orientation of the various waves. The 12-lead approach has the enormous and perhaps insurmountable advantage of being the established standard and any new electrode arrangement or graphic presentation proposed has to offer significant advantages in terms of additional information acquired or ease of acquisition to replace it.

The Utility of Electrocardiography

As noted earlier, the pattern of spread of excitation, especially through the ventricular mass, is complex. Any deflection, its magnitude and direction, on whatever lead merely represents the resultant of all electric effects during that instant, and without other information, it is not possible to decipher from the surface information alone taken from one lead individually or altogether what electric activity in which part of the heart contributed to it, or there is no unique solution to any particular electrocardiographic deflection. Be that as it may, by correlating ECG changes with findings in experimental preparations of one kind or another or with autopsy data, general inferences can be made about the electic forces generated by moving activation boundaries, realizing that only those that happen to escape concellation will have expression as a deflection on a particular lead at any instant in time.

The utility of electrocardiography is related to its unequivocal, unsurpassed, highly sensitive and specific value in the diagnosis of cardiac rhythms, including conduction disturbances, and to its empirical use in inferring the presence of a wide variety of metabolic or anatomic abnormalities of cardiac muscle that produce nonspecific alterations in depolarization (QRS complex) or repolarization (ST segment and T wave). The physiologic basis for some of these alterations in ECG pattern has been established, but for most the relationship of ECG change to disease remains empiric. The empirical approach lacks sensitivity and specificity because of the rather broad range of variability in both the normal and disease population, not to mention the obvious problem that the surface record can't discriminate unequivocally the location much less nature of a physiologic disturbance leading to the alteration in the surface record. Alterations in the T wave and ST segment are particularly noteworthy in this regard. Be that as it may, the clinical electrocardiogram has proved beyond doubt to be a most useful and valuable diagnostic adjunct.

ELECTROPHYSIOLOGY OF
CARDIAC RHYTHM DISTURBANCES

The property of automaticity provided by spontaneous pacemaker potential is not unique to SA node cells. It may not be the case that every cardiac cell has this potential, but there is no question that many do, particularly those of atria, AV node, and the specialized conduction system. The SA node ordinarily dominates impulse formation because it has the highest inherent pacemaking (diastolic depolarization) rate. The AV junction also has a higher rate than those of the cells of the specialized conduction system in the circumstances where either of these assume pacemaker function. Pacemaking function

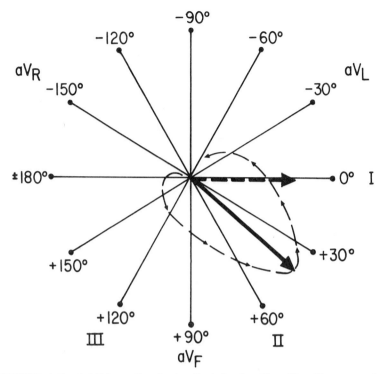

FIGURE 4–3 Addition of unipolar limb leads aV_R, aV_L, aV_F to standard leads, I, II, and III, provides six views of cardiac electric activity in the frontal plane at approximately (here plotted exactly) 30° increments starting at 3 o'clock positive in the clockwise and negative in the counterclockwise direction. Lead identification is placed on the positive hemisphere side of each lead. A representative QRS time–space loop is shown by the dotted arrowed line (this would be inscribed in about 80 msec) and its mean value shown as a solid arrow, which represents a QRS vector. (Similar loops and arrows could be represented for both the P and T waves). The broken arrow along the axis of lead I represents how the mean QRS vector would appear on that particular lead (a dominant positive wave). This could be done for each of the six leads. In actual practice the opposite process, deriving the mean QRS vector from the QRS deflections in any two (preferably separated by a wide angle) leads, is carried out.

originating outside the SA node is referred to as ectopic rhythm. The ectopically originating beat may be atrial, AV junctional, or ventricular; it can occur as an isolated event, sporadically, frequently, or exclusively; and it may be temporary, indefinite, or permanent. While ectopic beats are not necessarily associated with disease states (everyone probably has them at one time or another) when they occur sporadically (in the presence of normal sinus rhythm), there is no question that the cell or cells responsible for ectopic pacemaker activity are behaving unusually. If a higher pacemaker fails for any reason, the fact that there are other cells capable of assuming pacemaker function, albeit at a slower rate, reflects the degree of redundancy nature has designed into this vital function. For example, there are both congenital and acquired conditions wherein there is complete and permanent blockage of impulse transmission through the AV node (a condition termed complete heart block). In this circumstance, prior to the advent of artifical cardiac pacing, the patient's life obviously hinged on a lower (probably conduction system) focus assuming pacemaker function.

When the rate of an ectopic focus exceeds that of the SA node, it usually takes over the pacing function of the heart completely. If the focus is in or below the junction tissue, ventricular activation will coincide with or precede atrial and atrial contraction transport function will be lost. Ectopic supraventricular (atrial or nodal) pacemakers can fire as frequently as 200–240 times/min whereas ventricular tachyarrhythmias usually do not exceed 150/min. The limited capacity of the AV node to conduct impulses owing to its slow conduction velocity usually leads to some degree of physiologic AV node block, which provides protection against unduly rapid ventricular rates in atrial tachycardias. Ectopic pacemakers may not be subject to the powerful autonomic influences under which the SA node functions but their occurrence and rate are enhanced by depolarizing influences, such as sympathetic overactivity or administration of β-adrenergic drugs. Their suppression by pharmacologic agents generally occurs as a result of hyperpolarization of membranes and thereby reduction of automaticity.

While isolated, infrequent, or repetitive ectopic pacemaker activity originating in arial, junctional, or ventricular conducting tissue represents the most common mechanism for clinical rhythm disturbance, it is neither the only mechanism nor that causing the most dramatic arrhythmias. Another mechanism producing extra beats or tachyarrhythmias is based on the so-called reentry mechanism, originally referred to as the circus movement theory.

Reentry refers to the phenomenon wherein a depolarizing wave front gets channeled into an anatomic pathway wherein the potential for either isolated or repetitive circular conduction exists. Such pathways obviously must posses special electrophysiologic features for such circular non-extinguishing conduction to take place. Ordinarily a depolarizing wave encountering bifurcating double avenues for conduction will simply travel down both branches from the entry point, meet somewhere downstream, and continue on as a single depolarizing wavefront along receptive polarized pathways. The feasibility of reentry depends on the circular pathway permitting only unidirectional conduction, which means that counterdirectional conduction is blocked. The mechanism of unidirectional block remains a mystery but there is unequivocal evidence of its existence. Another condition requisite for non-extinguishing repetitive circular conduction is that the unidirectional depolarizing impulse continue to encounter repolarized tissue in its circular path so that it does not extinguish itself. This requires either that repolarization following depolarization be extra quick or that conduction be slowed. Considering prolonged cardiac action potential duration, the latter is what obtains and the two conditions together, unidirectional block and slow conduction, permit a circuit to be established, offshoots from which depolarize the remainder of the heart in repetitive fashion at a rate determined by the length of the anatomic pathway and the velocity of conduction in it. The term circus movement derives from the carousel-like nature of the electrical phenomenon.

There scarcely seems to be any doubt that reentry accounts for an atrial tachyarrhythmia known as atrial flutter. Reentry also accounts for certain premature beats whether single, multiple, or repetitive at various levels.

In atrial flutter the frequency of atrial depolarization averages about 300/min, about the maximum rate the adult human heart is capable (but not for long duration) of beating. The AV node usually is incapable of conducting impulses at such high frequencies, owing to prolonged refractoriness and slow conduction velocity. It therefore serves as a high-frequency cut-off filter conducting only some of these impulses in fixed or variable ratio (i.e., 2:1, 3:1, 4:1, or variable block).

While on the subject of AV node impulse conduction, it may be appropriate to interject here the role that this function plays in cardiac rhythm disturbances. As stated previously, the SA and AV nodes and atria are innervated by the vagus. Thus potentially there are two mechanisms for vagally-mediated heart rate slowing: reduced impulse formation in the SA node and blocked transmission. The latter is an example of atrioventricular block. AV block can be mild or severe and temporary or permanent. Mild or so-called first degree AV block consists merely of prolonged junctional conduction and is reflected in prolongation of the so-called PR interval without rhythm disturbance. The locus of the block can be anywhere between the SA node pacemaker and ventricular myocardium but in the vast majority of cases is in or below the AV node but proximal to the bifurcation of the His bundle. Rarely impulses may originate in the SA node, but either be delayed in emerging or partially or sporadically completely blocked. AV block beyond first degree is characterized by some degree of disparity between atrial and ventricular activation. In complete (3°) AV block disparity is complete, no atrioventricular relationship whatsoever. In 2° AV block it is something in between extending from varying prolongation of AV conduction and intermittent (not every beat) failure of conduction or fixed/variable AV ratio. Depression or failure of conduction presumably relate to alterations in membrane properties of certain cells in which either or both resting membrane or threshold potential are diminished (less negative).

Conduction system block beyond the point of His bundle arborization will not alter cardiac rhythm as long as one of the major branches is electrically intact. The depolarization of the ventricular mass in this instance will take a more circuitous route (the QRS wave will be distorted and prolonged) but each cell will receive the message each cycle. The further peripheral in the Purkinje system block occurs, the less the deviation from normal activation sequence of the ventricular mass and the less distortion and prolongation of the QRS complex.

To return to reentry as a mechanism for rhythm disturbance, it has also been invoked to explain perhaps the most dramatic of arrhythmias, atrial and ventricular fibrillation. In the ventricles it is dramatic because the rhythm is incompatible with effective cardiac contraction (i.e., the patient will die if it is not terminated or artificial perfusion is mandatory). Atrial fibrillation, while compatible with life even for prolonged periods, usually produces impressive irregularity of cardiac rhythm, due to variable AV block and sometimes very rapid heart rate when AV filtering function is diminished. The central notion concerning reentry in fibrillation is that rather than any fixed anatomic reentry pathway for repetitive stimulation, such as in atrial flutter, there are many simultaneous constantly changing ones. Considering the variability of action potential duration (APD) among cardiac cells normally present, if this variability were to be markedly increased for some reason there would be the potential for anatomically undefinable but multiple simultaneous physiologically traversable pathways throughout the cardiac mass for depolarization to stay alive without organized sequence because cells with short APD serve as pathways for and those with long APD sustain depolarization. Presumably this means that each cell stands a high chance of being depolarized (from different directions) again as soon as it repolarizes, but each would have its own frequency. This mechanism requires a certain minimum amount of cardiac tissue to be present, for small hearts of small animals cannot be fibrillated. Presumably this relates to the very short APD characteristic of small fast hearts and the markedly limited variability (disparity) of action potential duration of their individual cells. This mechanism does provide the possibility of self-extinction and such spontaneous termination is relatively common in atrial fibrillation but far less so with ventricular (larger muscle mass, longer APD, greater potential for disparity of APD).

The treatment of rhythm disturbances is beyond the scope of this presentation, but from what is known of their physiologic mechanism, the beneficial effects of various therapeutic inteventions, simple examples of which follow, should come as no surprise:

1. In the case of fibrillation (atrial or ventricular), delivery of a sudden large depolarizing current either directly to the heart or to the anterior chest wall with large electrodes (so-called DC defibrillation) depolarizes all cardiac cells simultaneously. This instantaneously restores order to chaos artificially. What is hoped for is that a regular pacemaker will then be able to resume function.

2. When the AV node blocks normal impulse transmission due to heightened vagal tone, the heart rate slows sometimes to the point of causing unconsciousness. It is a simple and effective matter to block vagal activity with the anticholinergic drug, atropine. If AV node transmission is temporarily depressed (such as may occur during certain phases of heart attacks) and atropine is ineffective or if the AV node is permanently disabled by disease, then it may be necessary to provide artificial ventricular pacing, either temporarily or permanently.

3. Occasionally, the simple maneuver of carotid sinus massage, which produces baroreceptor reflex vagal stimulation, is sufficient to convert an ectopic atrial tachycardia to sinus rhythm.

4. Pharmacologic agents that have been found to be effective in management of arrhythmias have one or another (or combinations) of the following properties: depression or stimulation of automaticity (hyperpolarize or depolarize cell membranes), depression or stimulation of conduction, and lengthening or shortening of action potential duration. Drugs such as digitalis have complex effects that vary with dosage including vagal stimulation, shortening of action potential duration, and enhancement of ectopic pacemaker activity. Drugs such as lidocaine, quinidine, procainamide, propranolol, and diphenylhydantoin suppress ectopic pacemaker activity, making them very useful in both prophylaxis and treatment of a variety of rhythm disturbances excluding those due to AV conduction block.

5
HEART MUSCLE

I discovered the following law concerning the dependence of the form of the isometric curve on the initial tension: The peaks (maxima) of the isometric curve rise with increasing initial tension (filling). (I call this part of the family of curves the first part.) Beyond a certain level of filling, the peaks decline (second part of the family of curves). The curves broaden steadily with increasing filling, and the area enclosed by the tension curve and the abscissa (the integral of tension) increases steadily, and does so even in the second part. Fick discovered the same law for skeletal muscle.

OTTO FRANK.
On the Dynamics of Cardiac Muscle. *Zeitschrift für Biologie* 32:370–447, 1895. Translated by Carleton B. Chapman and Eugene Wasserman. *Am. Heart J.* 58:282–317, 1959.

Of all the phenomenal things nature has to offer, the energy output of the heart must number among the more enduring. Large sums of money and much modern technology have been applied to development of an implantable artificial heart, and while progress has been made, the ultimate solution seems far off. The reason for pessimism relates to the difficulty of developing a durable, reliable, compact, lightweight, high-volume pump posing no problem in either energy availability or heat dissipation. If such efforts to date have accomplished nothing else, they have amply served to document what a remarkable biologic pump the heart is and what an amazing biologic engine (energy converter) heart muscle is. The average adult heart provides the body something in the order of 10,000 liters of blood flow per day, which, over the course of a lifetime, amounts to over 60 million gallons! This blood flows through vessels because of pressure gradients generated by cardiac contraction. The energy imparted to the blood by the heart is in both potential (pressure × volume) and kinetic (½ mass × average velocity squared) forms. Burton calculated that the heart performs about 2×10^9 foot-pounds of useful or external work during a lifetime, an amount sufficient to raise a 30-ton load to the top of Mount Everest (30,000 ft)! Prodigious as this may seem, it represents only a small fraction of total cardiac energy release (Chapter 6).

Every liquid transfer pump consists of at least two components: an energy source and a mechanism for transferring energy from the source to the medium being pumped. Biologic pumps are unique in that the two parts are one and the same: cardiac muscle in the case of the heart, the diaphragm and other respiratory muscles in the case of breathing, smooth muscle in the case of the urinary bladder, gastrointestinal tract, and gallbladder, and limb skeletal muscles in the case of venous return.

REVIEW OF SKELETAL MUSCLE AND
COMPARISON WITH CARDIAC MUSCLE PHYSIOLOGY

Skeletal and cardiac muscle are similar in structure and in the way that tension is developed in a functional unit, the sarcomere. However, they are quite dissimilar in the mechanism by which action potentials are generated and in action potential duration. Smooth muscle is different in many respects compared with both forms of striated muscle.

Every skeletal muscle cell is innervated by a terminal twig of a motor nerve. A group of muscle cells (100 or more) innervated by a single nerve fiber is called a motor unit, and a muscle bundle is comprised of one or more such units. A motor unit not only cannot contract in the absence of innervation, if innervation is permanently interrupted, the muscle unit atrophies or wastes (this is what happens in poliomyelitis because polio virus attacks and sometimes destroys the anterior horn cell in the spinal cord or medulla of the brain). The motor nerve terminal on the muscle fiber is called the neuromuscular junction or end plate; and electric activation of the muscle depends on a nerve action potential initiating the release of the chemical mediator acetylcholine (ACh) at the end plate. ACh, in turn, causes a localized electric disturbance in the muscle cell called the end-plate potential (EPP). As with so many nerve-mediated effects, calcium ion release is involved in the mechanism by which the nerve action potential is translated into ACh release from storage sites at the end plate region. The EPP depolarizes the muscle membrane to threshold level and an action potential is generated at the end-plate region that then spreads electrotonically along the membrane in all

directions with high velocity (5–10 m/sec). Since this happens simultaneously in all the cells of a motor unit, it is obvious why each unit
behaves functionally as though it were a single element.

Skeletal muscle action potentials are similar to those of nerve in
amplitude and are only modestly longer in duration. Because, for all
intents and purposes, each motor nerve action potential produces
one muscle action potential, the short duration of both provides the
possibility for high-frequency repetitive action potentials. However,
the mechanical process of contraction is relatively quite slow. Even in
so-called fast twitch muscle (e.g., eye muscle) there is a 7- to 8-msec
delay between the action potential and peak tension development. In
slow twitch muscles, such as those involved in maintenance of posture,
the delay may be as long as 90–120 msec. This means that electric
activation can be repeated many times while the mechanical event
related to each action potential is still in process, a circumstance that
allows summation of tension development. Thus, when the frequency
of action potentials is sufficiently high, maximum tension is developed, an effect that is called tetanus or a tetanic contraction. These
considerations of the voluntary motor system permit the exquisitely
fine gradation of force generated in a particular muscle; not only can
the number of motor units called into play be varied, the amount of
tension within each unit also can be graded depending on nerve stimulus frequency. Finally, by repeated exposure of muscle to voluntary
stress by work or physical conditioning/training, the mass, hence
strength, of muscle can be enhanced (hypertrophy or increased numbers of contractile fibrils/muscle cell). With hypertrophy, the range
of effort can be extended, ranging, for example, from the most gentle
of caresses to lifting several hundred pounds in athletic competition.

The morphologic similarities between skeletal and cardiac muscle
extend to the subcellular level. However, sarcoplasmic reticulum is
less extensive in cardiac muscle, whereas mitochondria are many
times more numerous. In both the functional subunit is the sarcomere, one of the series of elements containing the contractile proteins
connected end to end at each Z line (Figure 5–1). It has been demonstrated that when muscle contracts, the distance between two Z
lines is shortened as compared with that during relaxation (i.e., each
sarcomere shortens). The fact that the length of neither actin nor
myosin filaments varies during contraction, whereas the degree of
overlapping between them does, provides the foundation for the so-

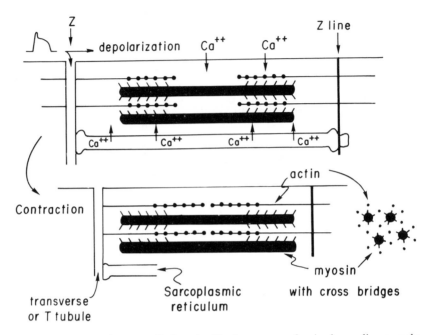

FIGURE 5–1 Diagram of a longitudinal segment of a single cardiac muscle sarcomere in the relaxed (upper) and contracted (lower) state depicting the sliding filament hypothesis wherein adjacent Z lines are brought closer together without change in length of actin or myosin filaments. Cross bridges and active sites producing filament sliding on myosin and actin, respectively, are shown as barbs and dots. Arrangement of filaments in cross section is shown at right indicating the large number of potential energy developing interaction sites. The plane of the section bisected a transverse tubule at the left Z line showing how membrane depolarization signal could lead to Ca^{++} release from SR storage sites. Not shown are many nearby mitochondria where ATP is generated and supplied to this mechanism for energy transduction (chemical to mechanical).

called sliding filament theory of the mechanism of muscle contraction. The idea is that muscle shortening results from an interaction between actin and myosin filaments that causes the actin filaments from adjacent Z lines to slide alongside the central myosin filaments and be drawn towards each other. Since actin filaments are tethered at their Z line ends, this movement results in adjacent Z lines being drawn together (i.e., shortening of the sarcomeres themselves). The force for this sliding motion is thought to develop between multiple so-called cross bridges on each myosin filament and active sites on surrounding (up to six) actin neighbors where biochemical energy in the form of ATP, produced in the mitochondria, is somehow translated to physical interactions that produce the sliding effect.

EXCITATION–CONTRACTION (EC) COUPLING

There is impressive evidence that calcium ion is essential for muscle contraction to take place. For example, it was demonstrated that injection of Ca^{++} directly into the interior of a muscle fiber with a micropipette produced contraction, whereas injections of other ions did not. It is now known that a Ca^{++} concentration of 10^{-6} M or more is required for contraction and relaxation depends on this concentration being lowered to 10^{-7}–10^{-8} M or less. The question then arises: Where does this Ca^{++} come from, how does it get there, what does it do, and how is the concentration lowered again so that relaxation can occur?

The continuous plasma membrane (sarcolemma) of the mammalian muscle cell has multiple invaginations in the region of the Z lines that extend into the interior of the cell. Since these intrusions are oriented perpendicularly to the long axis of the cell and are narrow, they are called transverse or T tubules. The so-called lateral cisternae or sacs of sarcoplasmic reticulum (SR) either abut on or are in close proximity to these T tubules. There is evidence that in skeletal muscle the SR serve as storage sites for Ca^{++}. The current concept is that either the action potential itself or, more likely, electrotonic current resulting therefrom, travels down the T tubules causing Ca^{++} in the nearby SR to be released. This Ca^{++} diffuses into the myofibril and when it reaches high enough concentration activates the actin–myosin cross linkages in each sarcomere. In cardiac muscle, this Ca^{++} release process perists throughout the duration of the action potential, whereas in skeletal muscle, because of the extensive SR, each action potential releases a burst of Ca^{++} ions adequate in amount to produce maximum twitch tension. This process can be repeated when the muscle membrane repolarizes and another nerve action potential comes along. Thus, during tetanus of skeletal muscle, a steady supply of Ca^{++} is made available to the contractile machinery by high-frequency repetitive action potentials. The highly developed SR in skeletal muscle provides plenty of Ca^{++} so that no other source is needed, but because there is less SR in cardiac muscle, apparently extracellular Ca^{++} (10^{-3} M) provides an important if not major additional source. Fish and amphibian cardiac muscle cells lack transverse tubules and have even less SR; muscle cells are much thinner and sparse myofibrils lie close to the surface. Therefore, in these species it is likely that most, if not all, Ca^{++} required for activation comes from extracellular fluid. There is evidence in skeletal muscle that suggests that active pumping (i.e., energy-consuming active transport) of Ca^{++} back into the SR, rather than passive diffusion, is necessary because the process requires ATP and can be blocked. It is not known what triggers this Ca^{++} pump, but if it exists in cardiac muscle its normal function is as important as the Ca^{++} release contraction mechanism.

The mechanism by which the action potential or its electrotonic extension triggers Ca^{++} release from the SR is not known, but whatever it is, recall that action potential-mediated calcium release is also involved in ACh release at the motor end plate in skeletal muscle; so too is norepinephrine release from sympathetic nerve endings. It may well be that these all share a common mechanism.

The mechanism by which Ca^{++} triggers the biochemical–physical process at the actin–myosin active sites also is not known, but the two possibilities include direct activation of the sites or Ca^{++}-mediated reversal of preexisting inhibition of the linkage mechanisms. Current evidence apparently favors the latter explanation. What physical process at the linkage sites (troponin–tropomyosin complex of actin and heavy meromyosin) produces the force for sliding of the thick and thin filaments is perhaps the greatest remaining mystery of all. There is no doubt that ATP generated in mitochondria through oxidative phosphorylation is the energy source for this mechanism.

MUSCLE MECHANICS

First established for skeletal muscle and found by Otto Frank to be equally applicable to cardiac muscle is the fact that, within limits, the amount of active tension a muscle can generate on shortening is directly related to the resting length of the muscle before contraction. That is, the more muscle is stretched beyond its passive unstretched length, the greater the tension it develops when it is stimulated to contract. As shown in Figure 5–2, however, this relationship is not

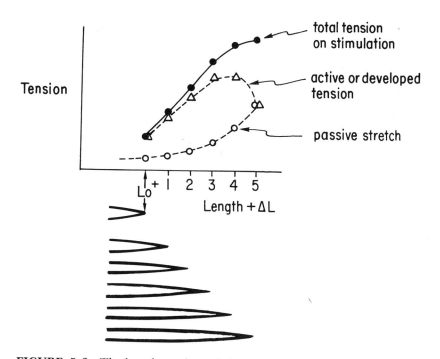

FIGURE 5–2   The length–tension relationship of skeletal and cardiac muscle. This intrinsic and fundamental property has its origin in energy generating sites in each sarcomere. The dotted, open circles line shows the tension produced in the muscle as a consequence of passive stretching produced by application of external force. At successive elongations of the muscle (as shown below) electrical stimulation results in the solid line-closed circles curve reflecting incremental total tension in the muscle. The active or developed tension in muscle is simply the total tension minus the passive tension at each length, or dotted line-open triangles curve. A family of such curves is shown in Figure 3–2. The main feature of this relationship is the progressive increments in active tension with increasing length up to a maximum beyond which it decreases. The length at which this peak developed tension occurs is assumed to be that which permits maximum actin-myosin interacting sites to participate in energy transduction. This relationship is the basis for the so-called Frank-Starling Law of the Heart, shown in Figure 6–5.

without limits. Stretching the resting unstimulated muscle itself produces increasing passive tension in the elastic components of the muscle. This increases markedly when the extensibility limit of the tissue is approached. In cardiac muscle, the magnitude of this passive tension with stretch is greater than it is in skeletal muscle. Beyond a certain optimal value, tension augmentation consequent upon contraction diminishes progressively to the point where contraction is incapable of producing an active tension increment over and above resting tension created by stretching. The rationale for this mechanism in skeletal muscle must have something to do with the mechanics of posture and locomotion. For the heart it represents an incredibly effective way of satisfying some very important requirements of the cardiovascular system.

The thick (myosin) filament is shorter than overall sarcomere length during contraction whereas the length of two actin filaments extending from adjacent Z lines is longer (if placed end to end) than sarcomere length during contraction but shorter than it is when the muscle is relaxed. Thus, not only is the degree of overlap between thick and thin filaments increased during contraction, thin filaments within each sarcomere may overlap each other. The resting length of muscle (sarcomeres) at which activation produces peak tension is thought to result from the degree of actin–myosin overlap which provides the maximum number of chemicophysical active sites (i.e., cross bridges). Resting lengths less or greater than this optimal length provide fewer sites, hence less tension development on activation of the system. The implication is clear that interaction points are limited to a limited segment of the overlapping ends of both filaments since the number of active sites diminishes with both greater as well as less than optimal overlap.

As you might predict, skeletal muscle is tethered at or near a resting length that provides maximal tension on activation (i.e., optimal overlap). Thus, motor units are in a position to achieve maximal tension at the onset of contraction when shortening begins to produce movement. To the extent that movement allows the ends (tendinous attachments) of the muscle to approximate, sarcomere length progressively diminishes as contraction proceeds. Thus, sarcomere length during successive action potentials gets shorter and shorter, overlap increases, and the amount of tension generated per twitch diminishes too. A contraction involving movement of a load is called an isotonic contraction because once the load starts moving, force is constant, and the lighter the load, the faster movement occurs. Contrarily, the greatest force is generated under the condition that movement of the load is prevented. To be sure, even when the ends of the muscle are fixed, sarcomeres do shorten (while series elastic components are stretched), but the degree of sliding is kept to a minimum and repetitive action potentials producing tetanus find the filaments nearest their optimal degree of overlap for maximum tension development. This is called an isometric contraction.

The two properties of skeletal muscle, the ability to produce tension or force on the one hand and movement (measured as velocity) on the other, are quantitatively described by what is known as the force–velocity relation. Maximum tension is developed during tetanus against a load that cannot be moved (isometric contraction) and maximum (theoretical) velocity, obtained by extrapolation, is developed at the beginning of a contraction where there is no load at all (so-called V_{max}). This turns out to be a hyperbolic relationship described by the Hill equation (after A.V. Hill, the Nobel prize-winning muscle physiologist):

$$(F + a) v = (F_0 + F) b$$

where a and b are constants, F = force, F_0 = maximum isometric force at tetanus.

While the force–velocity relationship adequately characterizes the mechanic properties of skeletal muscle contraction, there is no agreement as to the best descriptors of cardiac muscle mechanics. Force–velocity relationships have been obtained in cardiac muscle preparations, but the problems in this approach should be immediately obvious: Since cardiac muscle cannot be tetanized, there is no way to obtain F_0; thus, no way to extrapolate V_{max}. The ready availability of abundant Ca^{++} in skeletal SR provides for rapid maximal mechanical response to electric activation, but the long cardiac action potential duration and dependence on diffusion or extracellular Ca^{++} in addition to the limited amount available in the SR means that there is substantial delay (not to mention that associated with cell-to-cell transmission of the action potential) in reaching peak tension. This means that there will be significant time-dependence of any measurements one might wish to make or use. It also means that to the extent series and/or parallel elastic components and viscosity exist in the architecture of muscle fibers, one is more apt to get involved in their influences on mechanical behavior. But an even greater problem in cardiac muscle is that the strength of contraction is subject to alteration by factors other than length.

MYOCARDIAL CONTRACTILITY

If the length–tension relationship of both skeletal and cardiac muscle is explainable on the basis of the number of actin–myosin interaction sites which, in turn, relate to the degree of resting filament overlap, what is the mechanism of changes in cardiac contractile force that are known to be independent of length? Such changes (length-independent alterations in contractile force) are referred to as inotropic phenomena.

The first evidence of cardiac muscle inotropy was demonstrated in 1871 by Bowditch, who showed that changing stimulation frequency alone altered contractile force (with length held constant). This phenomenon was called treppe (staircase) because of the stepwise increments to the new steady-state level in tension development in response to a sudden increase in stimulus frequency. This is now referred to as the force–frequency relationship.

A second form of length-independent intrinsic alteration in cardiac contractility was discovered by Anrep in 1912. Working in Starling's laboratory and using the heart–lung preparation, Anrep found that when arterial pressure was suddenly increased, ventricular volume increased, as could be expected from Starling's law. However, within a short period of time, ventricular volume decreased toward or to the original volume despite the increased pressure load. Since cardiac output and heart rate were maintained constant (i.e., stroke volume constant), this meant that the ventricle was now performing greater external work without benefit of the length–tension effect (i.e., increased contractility). This Anrep effect has been observed in a variety of preparations since, but its mechanism remains obscure. Alterations in coronary blood flow have been excluded. There is no doubt, however, that the amount of pressure against which the ventricle pumps (nowadays referred to as afterload) is a length-independent determinant of contractility as is the case with treppe.

Bowditch demonstrated treppe in frog heart. Remember that frog cardiac muscle has no T tubules with little or no SR; therefore, extracellular Ca^{++} must diffuse into the fibers (which are thinner) during the very long action potentials characteristic of cold-blooded animals. During diastole, Ca^{++} passively diffuses out because there is no SR calcium pump. When stimulation frequency is increased, the period between action potentials shortens relatively more than action potential duration; hence, there is less time available for Ca^{++} efflux compared to influx. This leads to a progressive buildup in intracellular Ca^{++}, an effect that can also be achieved simply by increasing extracellular Na^+ or Ca^{++} concentration. The staircase phenomenon (or something closely akin to it) can be demonstrated in mammalian cardiac muscle, as well. This suggests that because of limited SR in cardiac muscle, the force of contraction is calcium concentration limited. In cardiac muscle, there is not enough Ca^{++} released during the action potential to remove inhibition from all potential active sites. Thus, presumably any intervention that enhances Ca^{++} entry during the action potential will increase force of contraction independent of length by activating more of the sites. Conversely, any intervention that limits buildup of intracellular calcium concentration during the action potential will decrease it. It has not been proven that interventions known to have positive and negative inotropic effects are mediated through the Ca^{++} effect, but neither has it been disproved. Conceptually, it is a reasonable starting point.

The question might logically be raised why Nature, in her presumed wisdom, would limit cardiac muscle contractile force by providing insufficient Ca^{++} to take advantage of the maximum available number of actin–myosin interaction sites? The answer is: she doesn't; at least when she desires not to. It has to do with functional reserve.

Remember that skeletal muscle force can be graded by the combination of at least two factors: number of motor units activated and nerve action potential frequency to those motor units. There is scarcely any necessity for an additional mechanism (excluding hypertrophy). Cardiac muscle has neither of these. How then is cardiac energy output graded to meet the wide latitude of demands placed on the heart?

The maximal energy demands on the heart can be prodigious. Imagine stroke volumes (Chapter 7) of 150 ml at heart rates approaching 200/min being ejected at a mean aortic pressure of 100 mm Hg in an athlete going flat out in intense competition. Compared to circumstances such as this, cardiac energy demands to provide resting body needs are trivial. Gradation of myocardial contractile force is an important element in the two-pronged cardiac response to such a wide range of demands, the other being heart rate.

To begin with, normal heart muscle is able to provide sedentary body needs at a resting sarcomere length less than the optimal length that provides maximal tension. Because submaximal amounts of Ca^{++} are provided by ordinary activation, the situation is one where not only are there fewer than maximum interaction sites, even those that are available are not all utilized because of Ca^{++} unavailability. Thus, only a fraction of tension-generating capabilities are used when demand is minimal. This means that there is an unused reserve that can be called into action through the mechanism either of greater (toward optimal) sarcomere length, increasing Ca^{++} availability, or both. In other words, the normal heart operates on the ascending limb of the length-tension relationship (Figure 5–2). Any effect that enhances diastolic filling, such as increased venous return, will automatically augment cardiac muscle energy output by increasing the number of potential interaction sites between the myofilaments (and vice versa) at any given level of Ca^{++} availability. Since the length–tension relationship has a descending limb, obviously extending sarcomere length beyond the optimal length would be self-defeating. However, the passive length–tension characteristics of normal cardiac muscle (i.e., it becomes much stiffer beyond optimal length) and the restraining effect of the pericardium are such as to guard against excessive passive stretch.

The second reserve mechanism consists of any and all factors that enhance Ca^{++} availability to the myofilaments thereby increasing the number of interactions participating in force development. It is worth emphasizing that the mechanism by which length-independent cardiac inotropic effects produce increased myocardial contractile force at any sarcomere length is unknown. While it is only speculation that all such positive inotropic effects will be found to be mediated through enhanced release and/or availability of Ca^{++} during the cardiac action potential, it is known that digitalis, the old, well-known, and much used cardiotonic, inhibits membrane Na^+–K^+ ATPase and leads to a net gain of intracellular Ca^{++}. There is also reason to believe that the most powerful inotropic effect of all provided by cardiac adrenergic stimulation (mediated by norepinephrine and epinephrine) may also involve the Ca^{++} mechanism. The inotropic interventions that affect the contractile force of cardiac muscle independent of length have no effect on skeletal muscle mechanics presumably because even under ordinary conditions the myofilaments are saturated with Ca^{++} during activation.

6

THE HEART AS A PUMP

... I am persuaded it will be found that the motion of the heart is as follows:

First of all the auricle contracts and in the course of its contraction throws the blood (which it contains in ample quantity as the head of the veins, the storehouse, and cistern of the blood), into the ventricles, which, being filled, the heart raises itself straightway, makes all its fibers tense, contracts the ventricles, and performs a beat, by which beat it immediately sends the blood supplied to it by the auricles into the arteries; the right ventricle sending its charge into the lungs by the vessel which is called vena arteriosa, but which in structure and function, and all things else, is an artery; the left ventricle sending its charge into the aorta, and through this by the arteries to the body at large.

WILLIAM HARVEY.
de motu cordis

The periodic nature of cardiac pumping results in repeating cycles of various time-varying phenomena, such as cardiac and intravascular pressures, chamber volumes, flow velocity, peripheral pulses, and heart sounds. These are depicted in Figure 6–1 and have particular relevance to clinical medicine not only because the manifestations of cardiovascular disease not uncommonly produce abnormalities in one or more of them, many are detectable by physical examination of the patient or by simple diagnostic technqiues. From the purely physiologic point of view, it should be obvious that all these cyclic phenomena are a consequence of the electric–chemical–mechanical cardiac mechanisms (initiation and spread of the electic impulse that produces an organized myocardial contraction) responsible for producing unidirectional flow in a valved muscular tube.

Timing of Events: Systole and Diastole

While the electrocardiogram is commonly used as a timing reference for cardiac events, other alternatives include heart sounds and venous or arterial pulses. It is necessary at the outset to define the two phases of the cardiac cycle, systole (systolic) and diastole (diastolic). Systole means contraction (Gr.), a mechanical event, ordinarily taken to mean of the ventricles as it pertains to the heart cycle. Thus, systole begins with the onset of ventricular contraction and ends when it is completed. The peak of the QRS deflection of the ECG is a reasonably sharp marker of the onset of ventricular systole, but the T wave lacks precision in defining the end of contraction. This imprecision is variously resolved by taking as a sharper end point of ventricular contraction: (1) the second heart sound, (2) the peak of venous V wave, (3) the incisura of aortic or central arterial pressure pulses, or (4) the return of intraventricular pressure to low levels, depending on which of these is available (these will be defined shortly). Diastole (Gr. dilatation), obviously, is the balance of the cycle relating to ventricular filling. Confusion has arisen from the use of the terms electric systole or electric diastole to denote the electric rather than mechanic processes of: (1) depolarization, its spread and repolarization, and (2) electric rest or inactivity. Another confusion arises from the equally ill-advised application of the same terms systole and diastole to compare (contraction or dilatation) artrial events. This is confusing because the atria contract during a part of ventricular diastole and fill during ventricular systole. It is reasonable, however, to apply systole and diastole to events in the arterial systems (systemic and pulmonic) because they are inseparably linked to equivalent ventricular mechanic events, even though there is slight offset in timing owing to the brief period of isovolumic contraction.

FIGURE 6–1 Chronologic interrelations among various cardiovascular events during a single cardiac cycle. Right heart events would be temporally and qualitatively similar but pressures would be about a sixth as high. The aortic root flow velocity curve at the top is tantamount to a volume flow curve assuming that aortic cross sectional area remains constant (flow = velocity × area). Features worthy of note include: (1) final LV filling volume increment provided by atrial contraction (atrial volume decreases reciprocally, of course, as is the case during all phases of the cardiac cycle), (2) onset of systole (ventricular contraction coincident with ECG R wave and S_1), (3) transient reversal of LV-aorta pressure gradient during the last phase of systole producing transient aortic flow reversal, aortic valve closure, and S_2, a good marker of the end of systole and (4) rapid part of ventricular emptying and filling S_3 occurring during first third of systolic ejection and diastolic filling, respectively.

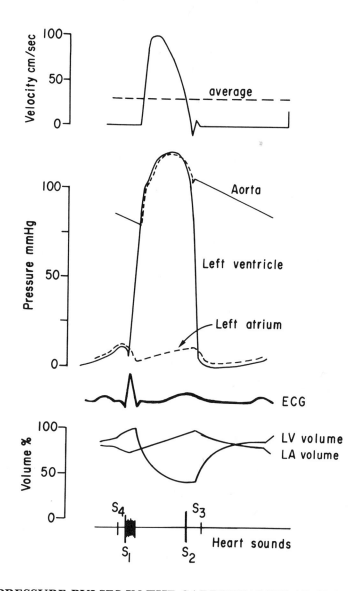

PRESSURE PULSES IN THE CARDIOVASCULAR SYSTEM

A pressure pulse is the contour or form of the graphic record of time-varying pressure in any heart chamber or blood vessel. The term must be distinguished from pulse pressure, which is the numerical arithmetic difference between peak systolic and minimum diastolic pressures, usually in an artery. Pressure pulses in the systemic and pulmonary circuits are qualitatively similar enough that a single description of the sequence of events suffices. Quantitatively, however, it is important to realize that in mammalian circulations left heart and vascular pressures are five- to sixfold higher than in the right.

VENTRICULAR PRESSURE AND VOLUME CHANGES

As the ventricular mass starts to contract, ventricular filling declerates and then abruptly ceases owing to the sudden reversal of the atrioventricular filling pressure gradient created by atrial contraction in the last phase of diastole. This reversal not only halts inflow, it closes the atrioventricular (AV) valves with such suddenness that a sound is generated, the first heart sound. The papillary muscles to which chordae tendineae of AV valves are attached are among early activated myocardium, and their early contraction provides the tension that prevents the ensuing rapidly rising intraventricular pressure from everting the leaflets during their closing. Once the leaflets coapt at their leading edges, the potential force for eversion suddenly diminishes because ventricular pressure on both sides of the coapted segment holds the leaflets together. The ventricular (end-diastolic) volume is at a maximum and it is trapped in a chamber, the tension in the wall of which rises steeply owing to contractile element shortening in the face of a virtually fixed incompressible volume (i.e., isometric contraction). The new energy in the form of tension created by the trillions of actin–myosin interaction sites is shared among all series elastic structures (this includes tension within the muscle fibers themselves, that outside muscle fibers but within the myocardium, and that outside the myocardium but part of the ventricular chamber, such as valves, chordae, membranous septum, etc.) and by the contained fluid itself in the form of pressure. This phase of cardiac contraction is called isovolumetric (isovolumic, for short) to convey the idea that ventricular volume is unchanged during it. The rate of intraventricular pressure rise is so rapid during isovolumic contraction that it quickly reaches the level in the outlet artery across the closed semilunar valve. The semilunar valves open when ventricular pressure exceeds the falling aortic root pressure. Once this happens, the new energy still being developed in the myofilaments is shared in additional ways and the rate of pressure rise slows. The contracting myocardium now encounters the elasticity (capacitance) of the blood vessels into which the blood is being ejected, the requirement to accelerate the motionless blood in the ventricle and the root of the aorta and the vascular resistance of the myriad pathways for egress. Thus, if contraction represents a source of new energy, vascular capacitance, inertia, and blood flow resistance represent sinks (collectively these are termed aortic impedance) into which energy can be stored or converted for useful purposes.

What all the foregoing means, as far as the ventricular pressure pulse is concerned, is that with opening of the semilunar valves two opposing effects are going on simultaneously. The fact that pressure continues to rise during early systole when maximum acceleration and ejection occur (potential to kinetic energy conversion), as well as stretching of vessel walls, means that contraction energy input exceeds its conversion and storage. The peak of ventricular and simultaneous aortic systolic pressure means input and loss have equalized. The decline in pressure beyond the peak means that the system expends energy faster than it is being added.

Ventricular volume begins diminishing as soon as the semilunar valve opens. It falls most rapidly during the first quarter of systole when ventricular contraction energy is maximal with respect to wall tension development and aortic input impedance is at its lowest. The rate of decline of ventricular volume falls off rapidly (more or less exponentially) as the rate of tension development diminishes progressively and aortic impedance reaches a peak. The rate of volume decrement during the last quarter of systole tapers to zero at aortic valve closure.

Recall that cardiac muscles develop tension almost as long as the action potential continues, but that action potential duration is variable (distributed) among the cells. Thus, while the onset of ventricular contraction may be more-or-less unified, relaxation is less so. When ventricular pressure begins to fall off rapidly towards the end of systole, the chamber itself becomes another potential flow sink. In fact, there is a momentary reversal of flow in the aortic root late in systole owing not only to the open aortic valve and falling ventricular pressure but also the widely patent coronary vessels. This reversal closes the semilunar valve abruptly. The energy stored in the stretched elastic tissues of the aorta and large arteries during systole now becomes an energy source for maintaining flow and pressure in the arterial system during diastole. Semilunar valve closure: (1) produces a small pressure notch on the arterial pressure pulse called the incisura, (2) eradicates the ventricular sink, and (3) produces the second heart sound. At this point ventricular volume is at its minimum or so-called end-systolic point, having ejected the stroke volume. Ventricular pressure then falls rapidly and isovolumically to the point where it is exceeded by existing atrial pressure whereupon the AV valves open again and diastole (ventricular filling) commences. The ventricles do not empty completely during systole. Rather, roughly 40% of the end-diastolic volume remains, the so-called residual or end-systolic volume. The ratio of the amount of blood ejected per beat, the stroke volume, to end-diastolic volume is termed the ejection fraction (EF = SV/EDV). Ejection fraction diminishes as a consequence of heart failure and is commonly used as an index of ventricular function, but unfortunately it is a rather insensitive barometer under resting conditions.

ATRIAL PRESSURE AND VOLUME CHANGES

The atria serve as passive conduits and reservoirs, except for the brief period (< 200 msec) at the end of ventricular diastole when, by timely contraction, they contribute an active role in terminal ventricular filling. The greater share of ventricular filling occurs passively as far as the atria are concerned and takes place during the early part of diastole. By contracting when the ventricles are almost filled, the atria add the final component of filling volume. Ventricular volume, of course, is directly related to sarcomere length; hence, myofilament overlap. Average or mean atrial pressure is determined by the diastolic or filling characteristics of the ventricle, blood volume, and venous tone. In normal man at rest, right atrial pressure is about zero (i.e., atmospheric) and left atrial pressure about 5 mm Hg, reflecting the difference in passive distensibility of the two ventricles, the left being stiffer.

The new energy resulting from atrial contraction (source) finds a number of sinks. Unlike the situation with onset of ventricular contraction where maximum intracavitary blood volume is immediately trapped, atrial blood volume at onset of contraction is approaching a minimum and then quickly reaches it because the open AV valves, as well as the veins, represent avenues for egress of blood. Thus, as shown in Figure 6–2, atrial pressure rise during contraction, the A

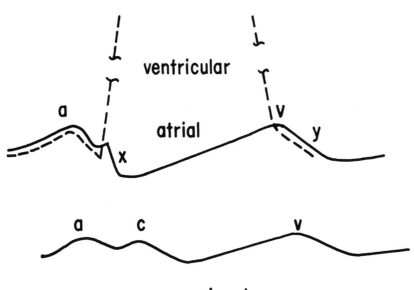

ventricular

atrial

a

v

x

y

a   c   v

jugular venous

FIGURE 6–2 Atrial (left and right qualitatively similar but quantitatively slightly different, left being higher) and systemic venous pressure pulses showing similarities and some differences. There is general timing offset; that is, delay in venous due to transmission delay between right atrium and neck vessels. The C or carotid (artery) impact wave is absent from the atrial (and presumably other noncervical veins) and the X descent (most prominent in left atrium due to ventricular stiffening and apex-directed force on the atrioventricular ring and valve apparatus) is locally dissipated and absent in the jugular pulse. The a wave reflects atrial contraction, the peak of the V wave maximum atrial filling, and Y descent rapid atrial emptying (see Figure 5–1).

wave, normally is trivial in magnitude, amounting to only a few mm Hg, while terminal ventricular filling occurs in preference to backflow into veins presumably because of momentum (blood is already flowing toward the ventricle). Then as ventricular contraction occurs, atrial pressure transiently (during isovolumic contraction) falls abruptly. This is explained by the chordae and valve leaflets being jerked toward the apex by the sudden stiffening of the heart (so-called descent of the cardiac base). This motion of the ventricles causes the apex of the ventricle to be thrust outward toward the chest wall producing a palpable (apical) pulse. Since venous flow was temporarily retarded, if not stopped, by atrial contraction, this jerk on the AV ring causes a slight increase in atrial capacity not accompanied by a volume increment; hence, the sharp transient pressure fall, which is called the X descent. Antegrade atrial filling from veins then commences during the remainder of ventricular systole. There is a passive rise in atrial volume called the V wave that crests at the point where pressure in the relaxing ventricle falls below atrial pressure and atrial emptying (ventricular filling) commences. The fall in atrial pressure which passively follows the declining atrial volume is called the Y descent, and it occurs primarily in early diastole when ventricular filling rate is more rapid. Atrial contraction, which completes diastole, then produces the small positive wave that is called the A wave.

HEART SOUNDS

Almost everyone learns that there are two sounds associated with each beat of the heart, "lub" and "dup." Actually, there are at least four; two lubs and two dups because of the series-connected pumps operating in parallel (i.e., side by side). Their virtually synchronous beating is what superimposes the lubs and the dups, but the trained ear of the discerning listener often is able to sort out the components because he knows how to take advantage of the limited asynchrony that exists. Graphic records (phonocardiograms) confirm the dual components of each heart sound. Thus, whatever it is that creates the sounds we can conclude that the same principles apply to each of the pumps.

Sound is a form of energy that results from vibration of a structure at a particular frequency and amplitude such that it imparts to the medium in which it exists compression and rarefaction of gas or liquid molecules that are then transmitted away from the source. Hearing involves the opposite of this process; that is, compression and rarefaction (sound) of air in the external auditory canal causing the tympanic membrane to vibrate. Whatever sound is produced has meaning only insofar as it is heard, recorded in a visual display for analysis, or is used to cleanse or destroy objects (sonication). Cyclic compression and rarefaction of gas or liquid molecules can originate in these media independent of a vibrating structure under certain conditions. For example, it has already been mentioned (Chapter 2) how turbulent flow or local formation of vortices may generate sound (a vortex or eddy is what happens to water on the back side of a canoe paddle when you pull it through stationary water; it is the wake behind a boat moving in the water or behind a rock sitting in a stream).

Thus, cardiovascular sounds can originate in structures, in blood, or in both. Whatever the origin, once developed the whole system participates and it is what gets transmitted in the medium at an energy level sufficient to be heard or recorded that is significant, for who knows (or cares) what vibrations or cyclic compressions and rarefactions that are occurring that are below the threshold of audibility or recordability. As electric energy is transmitted in the body medium (i.e., volume conductor), so too is sound energy. Both transmissions are complex because of variabilities and discontinuities of the medium. Each interface is a potential source of energy loss or alteration in the quality of the sound (damping, resonance, etc.). Whatever sound reaches the body surface, there is then the problem of getting it to the auditory cortex of the listener, and having heard it, there is the problem of interpreting or translating it into a form useful in communication to others. These latter considerations are beyond the scope of this presentation but they are pertinent to clinical medicine (i.e., auscultation in physical diagnosis). René Laënnec made a major contribution to medicine when he invented the stethoscope (1819), but he completely misinterpreted the significance of the heart sounds.

The original notion that heart sounds resulted from the clapping shut of atrioventricular (first sound) and semilunar (second sound) valves undoubtedly is oversimplified if not inaccurate. There seems little doubt that the second heart sound components (these are termed A_2 for aortic and P_2 for pulmonic) are coincident with closure of semilunar valves, but it is believed that it is the abruptness of the deceleration of blood that creates the vibrations rather than physical contact of the valve leaflets. The first heart sounds (M_1 and T_1) are much more complex. It is thought that abrupt deceleration again accounts for most of the sound because of the coincidence with atrioventricular valve closure, but in addition sudden tensing of the entire ventricular mass and sudden acceleration of both stroke volumes contribute components as well.

Several other sounds maybe heard in different subjects, under particular circumstances or in association with cardiac diseases, that substantiate beyond a doubt that valve closure is not necessary for sound generation. It is usually the case that such other sounds are softer (less amplitude or energy level) than ordinary heart sounds, but sometimes they are not. The third heart sound (S_3) coincides with rapid ventricular filling and it is also most likely due to a rapid deceleration transient. It is so prominent when the pericardium is thickened by disease that it is called a knock. The fourth heart sound (S_4) coincides with atrial contraction and probably represents another decleration transient. It is prominent when atrial contraction is forceful or terminal ventricular filling is impeded such as by either a hypertrophied or highly overfilled ventricle, both of which have restricted distensibility. In atrioventricular valve stenosis (narrowing of orifice due to fusion of leaflet commissures), abrupt crossover from a ventriculoatrial to an atrioventricular pressure difference often produces a heart sound called the opening snap that is audible following the second sound (but earlier than S_3). This might be thought of as being due to something akin to the popping or snapping of a sail subjected to a similar sudden reversal of wind direction. Dilatation of the aortic or pulmonary artery root or aortic or pulmonic valve stenosis may give rise to so-called systolic clicks, sounds occurring early during systolic ejection. The mechanism of such sounds is less clear.

Murmurs or bruits are sounds or noises of more prolonged duration; that is, they are characterized by persistent vibrations. They usually originate in the blood and may achieve energy levels sufficiently high that renders them palpable, as well as audible. Several mechanisms have been proposed to explain murmurs but among the more enduring are turbulence, whether generalized (flow velocity exceeding critical as defined by Reynolds) or localized in the form of vortex trails being shed at branching or obstruction points and cavitation (formation of micro gas bubbles).

Murmurs may be heard in perfectly normal people or signify specific disease processes. Either may be loud or soft, short or long, and sound like this or that. One of the important goals of clinical training is to learn the nuances of the characteristics of murmurs with respect to their location, radiation, character (or quality), timing, associated findings, response to maneuvers or interventions, etc., to decide which is which insofar as possible. The first step toward this goal is to understand the normal heart cycle and when and how the various sounds are produced.

CARDIAC ENERGETICS OR
HOW THE HEART PERFORMS WORK

Frank–Starling Law of the Heart

A physiologic discovery dealing with the heart pump, which is one of the historical landmarks in circulation physiology, is that of the Law of the Heart. In its simplest form, it might be stated thusly: Within limits, the more the heart is loaded or stretched during diastole, the more vigorously it contracts during systole. This is the so-called Frank–Starling Law of the Heart, and while it was enunciated 80 yr ago, few discoveries have withstood so well the test of time. We now know that the cardiac phenomenon Otto Frank (1895) discovered in the frog heart and that was rediscovered independently by Ernest Starling (1915) in mammalian heart is based on the length–tension relationship that had been discovered previously in skeletal muscle by Fick (1882) and Blix (1895). We also know that the phenomenon has a subcellular origin in each of the trillions of sarcomeres themselves and we even think we know what its molecular mechanism might be in terms of actin–myosin interaction sites. The road to this knowledge and understanding, however, was not smooth along its entire course. When deviations from the Frank–Starling law began to crop up in clinical observations, two options were suggested. The first was that the law simply was not applicable in intact animals. The second was that while the law was operative in the intact animal, it is overshadowed by other variables not normally functioning in a highly controlled and artificial nonphysiologic preparation, such as the heart–lung preparation in which it was discovered. The controversy has been satisfactorily resolved favoring the latter explanation during the past 30 yr on the basis of a series of brilliant studies by many investigators but especially those of Dr. Stanley Sarnoff and Dr. Robert Rushmer, which extended our understanding of cardiac function.

Frank and Starling depicted only a single curve as defining the relationship of external work as measured by pressure (Frank), flow, or both (Starling) to end-diastolic condition as measured by pressure (Frank) or volume (Starling). In retrospect, such curves demonstrate a low order of cardiac energy release, related, no doubt, to the unphysiologic preparations in which they were discovered. Sarnoff's

major contribution was the demonstration that the relationship for
any given heart was variable depending on the conditions of the experiment (he was careful to examine the two ventricles separately,
and he purposely imposed interventions that altered cardiac performance). He thereby introduced the concept of a family of ventricular function curves (Frank had demonstrated a family of pressure curves). Rushmer's contribution was his demonstration of the
extent and possible mechanisms by which extracardiac, especially
neural considerations, were superimposed on the intrinsic cardiac
work–end-diastolic condition relationship. The combination of these
insights provides our present understanding, which is that the normal
heart has a range of curves on which it is able to function, which one
at any moment it happens to be on depending on the interplay of all
factors that influence end-diastolic condition and cardiac contractile
state.

Pressure–Volume Loops and Ventricular Stroke Work

The relationship between simultaneous pressure and volume changes
that the ventricle undergoes during each heart cycle yields what is
known as a pressure–volume loop or diagram. Such a diagram is
illustrated in Figure 6–3 and it is instructive in providing not only a
graphic analysis of ventricular events during the cardiac cycle, but
also insight into the external work performance characteristics of the
ventricle. As will be discussed in subsequent chapters (16 and 18),
pressure volume loops also represent a useful way to depict how
ventricular function is altered under various physiologic and pathologic conditions.

The integral of pressure and volume change between end-diastole
and end-systole, $\int Pdv$, is stroke external work of the ventricle. The
kinetic or velocity component of ventricular work, ½ mass · velocity²,
is usually disregarded in consideration of external work because it
only comprises a few percent of total work during rest. (It should be
noted, however, that during severe exercise this might increase to
15–20%, which is certainly not negligible, and the kinetic component
may also be significant in disease states characterized by high flow
rates). The product of stroke work and heart rate per minute yields
ventricular work per minute. The relationship of energy of contraction to end-diastolic fiber length, of course, is the Frank–Starling one.
Therefore, relating the end-diastolic condition, whether end-diastolic
volume (V) or pressure (P), to P–V work provides an indication of

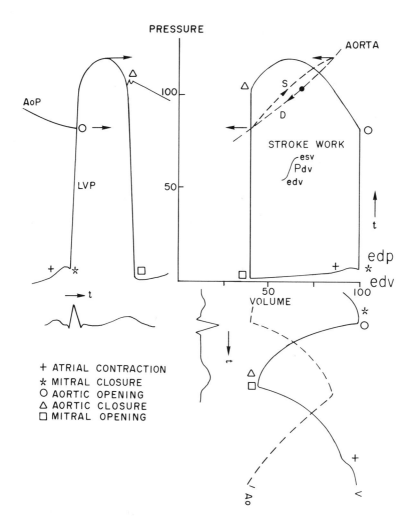

FIGURE 6–3 Ventricular and aortic pressure-volume loops (upper right) based on simultaneous left ventricular pressure (LVP) and volume (V in %) and aortic pressure (Ao P) and volume (Ao) relationships during a single cardiac cycle. ECG is shown as a time reference for both variables and various events are identified by symbols on each parameter as listed. A portion of aortic distensibility curve (P–V relationship) is shown with a closed circle separating systolic (S) from diastolic (D) P–V change. The narrow loop inscribed represents an illustration artifact, actual $P \cdot V$ changes take place along a single curve, the slope of which varies with distensibility. The area of the ventricular $P \cdot V$ loop is ventricular ($\int Pdv$) stroke work. The area of the gap at the bottom between the loop and the pressure baseline represents $P \cdot V$ work required by the right ventricle and left atrium to fill the left ventricle to its end-diastolic pressure (edp) and volume (edv) point.

how the ventricle is performing its function analogous to the way the length–tension relationship is a measure of how muscle works.

There is an interesting feature of ventricular and cardiac muscle work, highly pertinent to clinical medicine, that is appropriate to raise here. It is the important difference in the energy cost to muscle of developing and maintaining tension compared with that required to produce shortening (i.e., isometric-versus-isotonic contraction). That is to say when you grit your teeth, clench your fist, or hold a weight off the ground, you are doing no work in the physical sense, despite the fact muscles involved are generating force and consuming energy to produce the effect. Translated to the heart pump, this consideration relates to the distinction between the energy required to create and maintain wall tension that raises and maintains the pressure in blood during systole versus the energy required to eject the stroke volume. It has been known since Starling's day that the volume (ejection) dimension of work is accomplished with a great deal more efficiency than is the pressure.

Cardiac Efficiency

The efficiency of the heart pump can be defined the same way as that of any other machine. It is the ratio of the useful work output (i.e., $\int Pdv + \frac{1}{2} mv^2$) to the energy (i.e., caloric equivalent of oxygen consumption) consumed to produce that output. Cardiac efficiency is of low order-of-magnitude, usually only a few percent at rest, and no more than 10–15% during exercise. Thus, increasing stroke volume can be accomplished at less cost in myocardial oxygen consumption compared with increasing pressure by the same proportional amount. Low cardiac efficiency results from the fact that only a small part of the tension generated in the ventricular wall during contraction appears as useful external P–V work. The remainder represents the tension that has to be developed just to permit ejection to occur. Thus, as Burton has emphasized, the magnitude and rate of wall tension development more so than external P–V work reflects the total energy output of the heart.

According to the Laplace relationship ($T \propto Pr$), the factors that determine wall tension, T, are: (1) the magnitude of intraventricular pressure, P, (2) the end-diastolic volume of the chamber (which determines radii of curvature, r, during systole), and (3) duration of systole (time spent maintaining tension). Systolic duration, in turn, is directly related to heart rate. The geometry of ventricular chambers is far too complex to permit a simple description of the relationship between volume change and average radius of curvature change, but assuming a sphere (wherein volume = $4/3 \pi r^3$) radius is proportional to the cube root of volume. Therefore, because the Laplacian determinant of tension is radius rather than volume per se, a unit change in pressure has a greater effect on tension than does volume despite the fact that they have equal influence on P–V work.

Tension–Time Energy Component

The tension-versus-time curve of ventricular contraction, of course, cannot be measured directly the way pressure–time can. However, its qualitative time course can be predicted knowing the P–V and Laplace relationship as shown in Figure 6–4. During isovolumic contraction, average radius of curvature is at a maximum and it remains essentially fixed while P rises precipitously. Thus, tension must rise proportionally along the same time course. Once ejection begins, r decreases while P continues its ascent: at the point where the rates of both P increase and $k \sqrt[n]{v}$ decrease reach the same relative value, tension increase halts. It is likely, therefore, that the tension–time curve peaks and begins falling before peak-systolic pressure is reached. Once ventricular pressure starts declining, tension falls precipitously because P and r rapidly approach minima. The energy reflected in the area of the tension–time curve ($\int Tdt$) is the dominant component of total energy release during contraction. Increasing heart rate obviously multiplies this component almost in direct proportion whereas increasing stroke volume, especially if it can be accomplished by greater emptying compared to enhanced filling, has little effect on $\int Tdt$ because the base (time) is a function of heart rate while the height (tension) is more importantly determined by pressure than by volume. It is known that during positive inotropic interventions (such as occurs with exercise) the ventricle ejects more completely. Thus, stroke volume is maintained or even enhanced without greater end diastolic volume; the latter, in fact, may even decrease somewhat. This means that more P–V work is performed without greater tension development and probably explains increased cardiac efficiency noted during exercise.

The effect of myocardial length–tension-versus-inotropic state changes on the pressure–volume relationship are independent of one

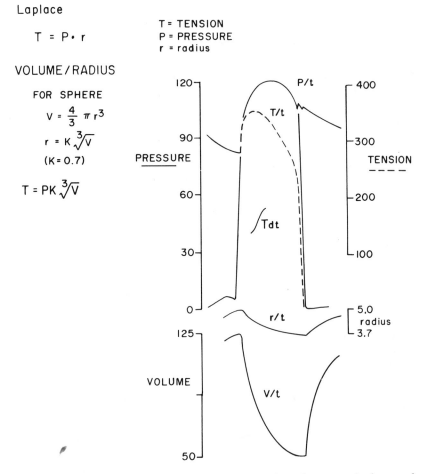

Laplace

$$T = P \cdot r$$

T = TENSION
P = PRESSURE
r = radius

VOLUME/RADIUS

FOR SPHERE

$$V = \frac{4}{3}\pi r^3$$

$$r = K\sqrt[3]{V}$$

(K = 0.7)

$$T = PK\sqrt[3]{V}$$

FIGURE 6–4 Derivation of approximate tension·time ventricular work from analysis of simultaneous left ventricle pressure/time (P/t) and volume/time (V/t) and assuming spherical ventricular chamber (an obviously invalid one) to derive radius/time (r/t). Dotted line is approximate tension with respect to time (T/t) and area within this curve ($\int$Tdt) is tension·time left ventricular energy, the dominant component of ventricular work.

another and critical assessment of ventricular function dictates that the role of each is either controlled or measured while the other is being evaluated. To the author's knowledge, no single measurable physiologic parameter has been identified to date that provides a measure of the length–tension relationship that is independent of inotropy, and conversely, none reflecting inotropic state that is independent of length–tension relationship. At any given inotropic state, increasing ventricular end-diastolic volume, such as by increasing venous return, produces greater P–V loop area; conversely, lesser ventricular diastolic filling the opposite. Whether the change in area will be reflected by alterations in pressure, stroke volume, or both depends on other factors. On the other hand, at any given degree of ventricular filling, a positive inotropic effect will be associated with greater, and a negative inotropic effect by smaller P–V loop area (Figure 6–5). Again, whether a particular dimension or both pressure and volume will change depends on external factors. The fact that the external work of the heart is only a small fraction of the total energy released during contraction means that this approach to analysis of ventricular function is rather insensitive.

To make an analogy with something perhaps more familiar, consider how the performance of an automobile engine is evaluated. The power output of an internal combustion engine is proportional to the engine revolution frequency (revolutions per minute or rpm). Gasoline consumption is also proportional to rpm; thus, power and fuel utilization are directly related. The performance of an automobile is gauged by how fast it will go, how rapidly it accelerates, how easily it climbs hills, what gear you have to use to climb a particular hill, etc. These are all measures of the rate of external work (i.e., power) produced by the engine. If you had an engine rpm indicator (some cars are equipped with such a device known as a tachometer), you would be able to discern the relationship between engine rpm and power (speed, etc.). You actually get an indirect sense of this from the sound of the engine and how much pressure you apply to the accelerator. But the most sensitive way to determine engine performance is to measure how much fuel is consumed (total energy input) relative to a particular rate of external work. (This is where the lesson of engine inefficiency is quickly learned.) To relate this to the heart, P–V work/end-diastolic condition (i.e., Frank–Starling relationship) is analogous to power output/rpm relationship and myocardial oxygen utilization to engine fuel consumption. The fact that only a small fraction of O_2 consumed and gasoline burned emerges as useful external work (the balance appears as myocardial wall tension heat in the case of the heart and heat in the case of engines) means that evaluating performance by external work output in relationship to

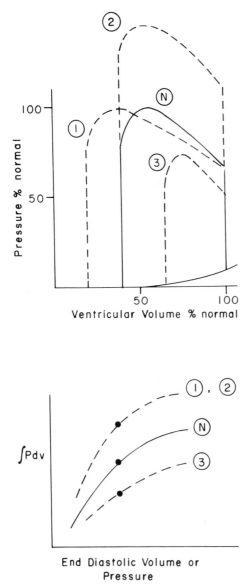

FIGURE 6–5

Frank–Starling–Sarnoff ventricular function relationship. In the upper figure several pressure–volume loops are shown starting at the same end-diastolic condition (100% volume, 10% pressure). N is the normal curve with a stroke volume (SV) and ejection fraction (EF) of 60%. Curve 1 shows increased pressure volume work (loop area) due to SV and EF of 80%. Curve 2 shows increased area owing to normal SV ejected at higher (145%) systolic pressure. Curve 3 shows diminished area due to both small SV and low-systolic pressure. When loop areas, $\int$ Pdv, or ventricular stroke work is plotted against the common end diastolic condition, the relationship depicted in the lower figure may be derived. The normal stroke work–end–diastolic condition relationship is a point (closed circle) on a continuum shown by the solid line, N. The increased stroke work (area) of loops 1 and 2 plots directly above the normal point and is, therefore, on a different ventricular function curve, 1, 2, reflecting increased contractility since ejection started from the same end diastolic condition (i.e., sarcomere length). Loop area 3, on the other hand, plots below on dotted curve 3 indicating depressed ventricular function, negative inotropy or heart failure.

indirect measures of input such as rpm or end-diastolic volume rather than total energy consumption will lack sensitivity (Figure 6–6).

If engine power/rpm is analogous to the Frank–Starling relationship, the question can be raised as to whether an analogy to cardiac inotropy exists. Recall that a change in cardiac inotropic state can be either positive or negative (improved or diminished force of contrac-

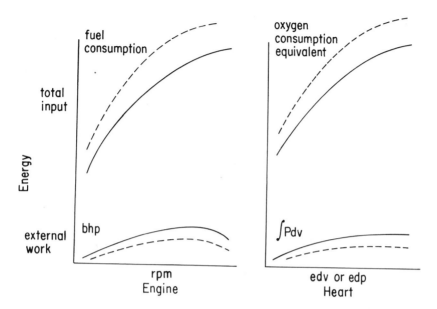

FIGURE 6–6 Comparison of internal combustion engine (left) and heart (right) in terms of useful or external work output (expressed as brake horsepower, bhp, and stroke work, $\int$ Pdv, respectively) compared to total energy utilization or requirement to produce that work, expressed as fuel or O_2 consumption, respectively. Note the same low degree of efficiency of both energy transducers. Failure of the engine or heart (dotted lines) is characterized by depressed external work output, enhanced energy consumption, or both (i.e., depressed efficiency).

tion at any fiber length) and that some external intervention usually is involved (sympathetic stimulation, hypoxia, etc.) in producing the change. Similarly, engine performance (power at any rpm) can undergo change depending on purposeful or inadvertent interventions (excluding modification of the moving parts of the engine itself). For example, changing fuel quality (so-called octane rating), carburation, ignition, or exhaust can have marked effects on the power/rpm relationship in either direction. Modification of the moving parts of an engine (such as by machining parts to closer tolerances—this is called blue-printing—or by chronic wear and tear) can have even more striking effects on performance without change in engine dimensions or design. Thus, auto racing enthusiasts utilize every possible means of maximizing the power output of an engine of given size by such positive inotropic interventions. In so doing they are only following the lead of nature in providing maximum flexibility and efficiency in engine function.

7
CARDIAC OUTPUT

Let us assume either arbitrarily or from experiment, the quantity of blood which the left ventricle of the heart will contain when distended to be, say two ounces, three ounces, one ounce and a half—in the dead body I have found it to hold upwards of two ounces. Let us assume further, how much less the heart will hold in the contracted than in the dilated state; and how much blood it will project into the aorta upon each contraction;—and all the world allows that with the systole something is always projected, a necessary consequence demonstrated in the third chapter, and obvious from the structure of the valves; and let us suppose as approaching the truth that the fourth, or fifth, or sixth, or even but the eighth part of its charge is thrown into the artery at each contraction; this would give either half an ounce, or three drachms, or one drachm of blood as propelled by the heart at each pulse into the aorta; which quantity, by reason of the valves at the root of the vessel, can by no means return into the ventricle. Now, in the course of half an hour, the heart will have made more than one thousand beats, in some as many as two, three, and even four thousand. Multiplying the number of drachms propelled by the number of pulses, we shall have either one thousand half-ounces, or one thousand times three drachms, or a like proportional quantity of blood, according to the amount which we assume as propelled with each stroke of the heart, sent from this organ into the artery; a larger quantity in every case than is contained in the whole body! . . .

WILLIAM HARVEY.
de motu cordis

The cardiac output is the amount or volume of blood pumped by the heart per minute and it is regulated to provide the internal milieu of the body with an adequate oxygen supply. How this is accomplished in the face of the incredible variation in conditions to which the body is subjected is a complex phenomenon that in mammalian circulation interestingly enough is based more on sensing and regulating blood pressure rather than oxygen delivery. The cardiac output (CO), as Harvey indicated, has two physiologic components, stroke volume (SV) and heart rate (HR):

$$CO = SV \times HR.$$

This simple equation states that regulation of cardiac output ultimately will be achieved through adjustment in either or both its components. As they are extemely important physiologic variables, it is appropriate to consider them individually.

HEART RATE

The rate of the heart beat theoretically can be altered by isolated changes of three variables of sinoatrial (SA) node cells (see Figure 3–3): (1) threshold potential (TP); that level at which sudden rapid membrane depolarization occurs and a propagated wave established. The more negative TP is the faster the heart rate and vice versa. (2) Membrane resting potential (MRP); the less negative MRP, the faster the rate and vice versa. (3) The slope or rate of slow diastolic depolarization or pacemaker potential (PP); the faster this rate, the faster the HR and vice versa. The available evidence suggests that changes in MRP and rate of PP account for most heart frequency changes and these are mediated by the autonomic nervous system.

CONTROL OF HEART RATE

The mammalian heart is richly innervated by the two divisions of the autonomic nervous system for two different but physiologically linked purposes: to produce changes in heart rate (chronotropy) and changes in heart contractile force (inotropy). Of these two divisions, the parasympathetic (vagus) is the more primitive because in many lower vertebrates heart rate changes occur only as a consequence of changing vagal tonus. In most mammals, including man, both right and left vagus nerves send branches to the heart that are distributed mainly to the SA and atrioventricular (AV) nodes and to atrial muscle. Both afferent and efferent vagal cardiac fibers have been identified, but our concern here is with efferent vagal innervation. Vagal stimulation slows the heart rate, delays or even blocks impulse transmission through the AV node, and diminishes the force of contraction of the atria.

Postganglionic sympathetic nerves from the superior, middle, and inferior cervical and upper thoracic ganglia form a rich cardiac plexus that is widely distributed to atrial and ventricular muscle, coronary vessels and to the SA and VA nodes. Stimulation of cardiac sympathetic nerves increases heart rate and force of cardiac contraction and dilates coronary vessels.

The autonomic control of the heart rate is best described by a simple relationship:

$$HR\alpha\frac{\text{Sympathetic stimulation}}{\text{Vagal stimulation}}\text{ of SA node}$$

This equation states that the sinoatrial node cells are under the tonic influence of competing forces that tend to speed or slow heart frequency. Reciprocal in their effect, enhancement of sympathetic stimulation, and diminution of vagal stimulation both speed the heart and vice versa. Heart rate increases (tachycardia) are explicable on the basis of inhibition of tonic vagal stimulation, sympathetic stimulation, or both effects acting concurrently. Heart rate slowing (bradycardia) usually is due to heightened vagal stimulation. An analogy might be made of a room the temperature of which was the resultant of both the heater (sympathetics) and air conditioner (vagus) operating simultaneously, a situation in which room temperature can be changed more than one way.

It is known that SA node slowing consequent upon vagal-mediated acetylcholine release results from increased membrane permeability to potassium ion. This has the effect of increasing MRP (more negative) and decreasing the slope of PP. It is not so clearly established whether the sympathetic effect on PP is achieved through increased sodium permeability, decreased K^+ permeability or a combination of these or other effects.

Now that the mechanisms regulating the heart rate have been considered, it is worthwhile to analyze what happens to cardiac output when the heart rate alone is experimentally manipulated: It is a simple matter in an anesthetized, open-chested dog to crush the SA node (which results in a slower heart rate from a junctional pacemaker) and pace the heart with an artificial stimulator. The interesting result of such a simple experiment is that within a rather wide range of heart rates above and below normal, cardiac output remains relatively constant and only at the extremes of slow (bradycardia) and fast (tachycardia) rates does the cardiac output fall. This is an important observation because the heart intrinsically is not a constant stroke pump, the output of which can be varied merely by changing the rate as in the case with mechanical pumps. It also tells us that there is a mechanism that adjusts the stroke volume inversely by just the right amount such that within particular limits, as long as the oxygen de-

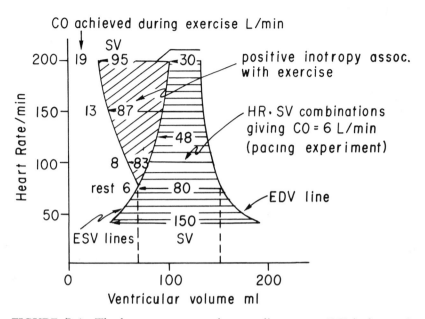

FIGURE 7-1 The heart as a pump where cardiac output (CO) is the product of heart rate (HR) on the ordinate and stroke volume (SV), which is the difference between end-diastolic (EDV) and end-systolic (ESV) ventricular volumes, on the abscissa. The dotted lines show approximate normal resting condition. HR = 75, SV = 80, CO = 6 L/min. In the resting state increasing or decreasing heart rate is associated with little change in cardiac output; thus SV decreases or increases, respectively, inversely. This is shown by the horizontally hatched area narrowing (smaller SV) with fast and widening with slow heart rates. EDV diminishes with rapid and increases with slow rates because of altered filling; this automatically alters ESV according to the Frank–Starling relationship. Cardiac output associated with exercise clearly involves other effects. In the untrained individual output is increased during exercise by SV being maintained or even increased somewhat (80 → 95) despite higher heart rate permitting CO to increase (6 → 19). This is mediated by a positive inotropic effect on the heart from adrenergic stimulation, as shown in Figure 6–2 (see Chapter 12), and increased venous return from the effect of the skeletal muscle pump (see Chapter 10).

mand of the body does not change, CO does not change either (Figure 7–1). This means that observed changes in CO such as during excitement or exercise must be achieved by effects independent of or in addition to heart rate variation. It would be a mistake, however, to infer from this experiment that heart rate control is of no physiologic importance, for as we shall soon see, it is very important (remember that in our simple experiment oxygen consumption was purposely held constant).

It is now appropriate to consider the other component of cardiac output, stroke volume.

STROKE VOLUME

Stroke volume (SV) is the amount of blood the heart expels with each beat. It is the difference between the volume of blood in the heart when it is full as compared to that following ejection. These are known as the end-diastolic (EDV) and end-systolic (or residual) volumes (ESV), respectively

$$SV = EDV - ESV .$$

Obviously, alterations in stroke volume can result from changes in either or both its component volumes.

Before considering the regulation of stroke volume, there is the fundamental issue of what determines the size of the normal heart, for it should be obvious that heart size by itself would be a critical determinant of stroke volume. Intuition would lead one to predict that the size, mass or pumping capacity of the heart varies with the number and magnitude of demands placed on it. The demands include: size of the animal, gravitational forces, other environmental conditions, and habits of the species, expecially activity. Considering only mammalian species, it is obvious that these demands can be extremely variable. For example, reflect on the rather special circumstances of the whale (size), the giraffe (effect of gravity), llama (altitude), and the race horse (effort). The interesting thing is that despite this variability, hearts of mammalian species eject a stroke volume during rest that is a remarkably uniform fraction of the end-diastolic volume (so-called ejection fraction) of about 60%. Thus, resting stroke volume in different species basically is determined by ventricular end diastolic volume which is primarily a function of heart size. Heart rate, of course, varies tremendously from species to species and, in general, it inversely relates to end-diastolic volume; the smaller the latter, the faster the resting heart rate. Another way of saying this is small hearts beat faster. Thus, a 600-kg whale heart beats 15 times during the same minute that a mouse heart might beat 300 or a hummingbird heart 1000 times. The exact physiologic mechanisms underlying these species differences in resting heart rate are not clear, but differences in response to or levels of thyroid hormone may be involved since metabolic rate is inversely proportional to body mass.

CONTROL OF STROKE VOLUME

In lower forms the heart consists merely of a few cardiac muscle fibers along a tube that in contracting create a sloshing undirected agitation of the contained blood. With phylogentic development, flow is not only directed by the presence of valves, it becomes circular, in lower forms with a single pumping chamber and in higher forms with two. Two chambered systems, in turn, are at first interconnected, but in highly developed mammals are completely separated.

The biologic survival value of the length–tension relationship of cardiac muscle is that it provides primitive circulatory systems a built-in or automatic mechanism for the heart to adjust its energy output to its input conditions, such that it can satisfy requirements placed on it without the necessity for a complex extracardiac control mechanism. By putting out more when it receives more (which also means, of course, that it receives more when it puts out more), increased flow requirements of locomotion (or whatever) can be met in lower forms without any additional mechanism such as heart rate adjustments or external nervous and/or hormonal systems. The fact is, however, that during the course of phylogenetic development a mechanism evolved in the aneural hearts of lower forms wherein distention of a cardiac reservoir chamber (sinus venosus) leads to increased frequency, as well as increased contractile force. It should be emphasized that in a system where the loading condition determines rate and/or contractile force, peripherally mediated effects on return of venous blood to the heart are paramount in initiating alterations in cardiac output, and effects such as that of skeletal muscle contractions on venous blood flow are well documented.

The length–tension relationship of cardiac muscle and the predominantly passive nature of ventricular filling provide one of the mechanisms for the observed results of the experiment cited earlier wherein artificially controlled heart rate changes within certain limits are not associated with cardiac output changes as long as oxygen consumption is held constant. The heart has a built-in mechanism for adjusting the duration of electric depolarization inversely to heart rate. Contraction duration (mechanic systole) in turn is tied to the duration of electric depolarization. Thus, as heart rate increases, mechanic systole of each beat shortens and tension generation diminishes accordingly. However, because there are more beats per unit time, the duration of systole/minute doesn't increase as much as would be the case if the duration of systole per beat were fixed. It goes without saying that diastolic (filling) duration per minute decreases as heart rate increases. Assuming no change in the pressure gradients for venous return and passive ventricular filling, shorter filling time per beat and per minute translates to less diastolic filling. According to the length–tension relationship this means a smaller stroke volume.

The other mechanism that limits cardiac output changes when heart rate alone is manipulated is the collapsibility of the venous reservoir (i.e., right atrium and vena cavae). If more blood is pumped out of the reservoir than is feeding into it, it merely collapses. This translates to lower pressure and less right ventricular filling. Thus, venous return plays a permissive role in cardiac output regulation, preventing nonphysiologic tachycardias (of which there are many varieties) from creating a situation of runaway cardiac output.

Slowing the heart rate should have opposite effects, but in the normal heart in this case, the relatively stiff passive distensibility characteristics of cardiac muscle and the pericardium limit diastolic filling even though duration is prolonged. In this situation the active part of ventricular filling owing to atrial contraction becomes important, and because atrial cardiac muscle also obeys the Frank–Starling relationship, atrial contraction associated with extended atrial filling would be stronger. It is well established that if an unphysiologically slow heart rate is experimentally imposed on a normal animal for a prolonged period (such as by destroying the atrioventricular node, which produces a condition called complete heart block), stroke volume gradually increases from that which obtained acutely at the time heart rate was slowed. This results from both greater ventricular filling and emptying. In fact, progressive compensatory increase in end-diastolic volume (and heart size) is such that despite markedly restricted heart rates, resting cardiac output usually returns to normal. Because these changes occur without marked increase in ventricular filling (and atrial and venous) pressures even though ventricular mass and volume increase, it is clear that increased passive ventricular distensibility is an important component of this compensatory phenomenon.

In the rather simple experiment of artificial cardiac pacing previously outlined, the animal at least had intact cardiovascular reflexes for factors other than nerve-mediated rate control (i.e., the sympathetic nerves to the heart were still intact). Incredibly, it has been demonstrated that racing greyhounds with totally denervated hearts not only can survive, their maximum exercise capacity and performance tested by stopwatch is only slightly blunted! Thus, as important as nerve-mediated adjustments in cadiac function are, as we shall see, it is clear that they do not represent the only line of defense. The Frank–Starling or length–tension Law of the Heart, primitive though it might be, is a fundamentally important one.

AUTONOMIC NERVOUS SYSTEM
AND CARDIAC OUTPUT REGULATION

Phylogenetic sophistication of the cardiovascular system basically related to developments that permitted increased oxygen supply to skeletal muscle without sacrificing, except for transient periods, the requirements of other tissues. Indeed, these adaptions along with the development of lungs and a protective integument served the permissive role that allowed organisms to leave the sea and range over the land. The components of progressive sophistication of the cardiovascular system include: (1) separating the system for obtaining oxygen from and eliminating carbon dioxide to the environment (pulmonary circulation) from that for transporting these gases to and from the body (systemic circulation), (2) control of heart rate, (3) control of the force of contraction independent of the length–tension mechanism, and (4) control of the distribution of the cardiac output by means of control of the peripheral blood vessels with respect to resistance (arterioles) and capacity (veins). The last three are achieved by the autonomic nervous system. In the discussion that follows focus will be on item 3; items 2 and 4 are covered in Chapter 12.

It was pointed out previously that stimulation of the sympathetic nerves to the heart produces three effects: higher heart rate, increased force of cardiac muscle contraction, and dilatation of coronary arteries. It should be apparent on intuitive grounds alone that these effects might combine to produce an increase in cardiac output and this indeed is the case.

Thus, the primitive length–tension relationship, a fundamental and intrinsic property of cardiac muscle and of the heart (i.e., Frank–Starling), is modulated by extracardiac factors. The number, variety, and power of these varies from species to species but seem to be highly developed in all mammals.

The development of sympathetic innervation of the heart represented a major achievement of nature. It provided aerobic organisms with a huge oxygen transport reserve that could be called on instantaneously. The sympathetic nervous system is often referred to as the fight or flight system. What is meant by this is that it is a system that automatically produces the visceral responses necessary for maximal motor capability to fight or flee. In this context, the cardiac response obviously is of major importance.

We noted earlier that artificially increasing heart rate alone had little effect on cardiac output because of a proportional decrement in stroke volume that resulted in the product of the two variables remaining constant. This was explained on the grounds of: (1) the lack of change in venous return (i.e., the heart can't pump out more blood than it receives), (2) the shortened period for diastolic filling of the ventricle per beat and per minute, and (3) the effect of the above two factors on the Frank–Starling mechanism (i.e., less filling, less output).

In lower forms, augmentation of cardiac output involves rapid adjustments in venous return not necessarily tied to a prior increase in cardiac output. This is equally important in higher vertebrates but, in addition, there is a mechanism for stroke volume to be maintained despite shorter filling time and diminished diastolic loading. Cardiac sympathetic nerve stimulation and increased circulating levels of plasma epinephrine resulting from adrenal medullary stimulation combine to produce what is known as a positive inotropic effect on the heart.

CARDIAC SYMPATHETIC INNERVATION AND STROKE VOLUME CONTROL

Unlike the length–tension relationship, which is an intrinsic property of heart muscle, inotropy involves a change in the chemical environment in which the heart muscle fibers function. In other words, an external intervention is required, which in one way or another, alters the contractile machinery independent of length. We now know of several interventions that enhance or depress the energy liberated during contraction. The former are referred to as positive and the latter negative inotropic agents. In addition to sympathetic stimulation, dopamine, norepinephrine, epinephrine, and calcium ion, which are endogenous physiologic positive inotropic agents, there are a host of sympathomimetic (sympathetic-like) drugs and digitalis. On the negative side are factors such as myocardial hypoxia (low oxygen), depressed Ca^{++} levels, toxic levels of most central nervous system depressant drugs, and abolition of physiologic sympathetic tone.

An inotropic effect can be demonstrated in preparations ranging from isolated muscle in a bath (Figure 3–2) all the way to the intact animal as long as the loading condition (stretch) can be controlled or measured and one has some way of quantifying the force of contraction, preferably both before and during the intervention under study. What these types of studies show is that positive inotropic interventions are characterized by augmented energy output of the heart, however it is measured, at any given diastolic fiber length compared to that produced in the absence of the intervention; negative inotropy the opposite (Figure 6–5).

It should be clear by now how the heart, armed with its sympathetic innervation, is capable of such a wide range of output. Tachycardia, as we have seen, is accomplished by withdrawal of tonic vagal depressor tone coupled with sympathetic stimulation of the SA node. The widespread distribution of sympathetic nerves to both atrial and ventricular musculature as well as coronary vessels enhances the strength (and speed) of contraction of both chambers while at the same time myocardial blood supply is increased. The increased strength of atrial contraction due to sympathetic stimulation contributes significantly to ventricular filling during tachycardia, adding, by means of the length–tension relationship, another component to ventricular contraction already enhanced by positive inotropy. Thus, instead of falling, stroke volume is maintained in the face of tachycardia, and in this circumstance cardiac output can increase in direct proportion to the increase in heart rate the same way that fixed-stroke mechanical pumps work. This effect is shown in Figures 7–1 and 7–2.

What about those racing greyhounds with denervated hearts? What about patients with transplanted hearts or those taking drugs such as reserpine and propranolol that deplete catecholamines and

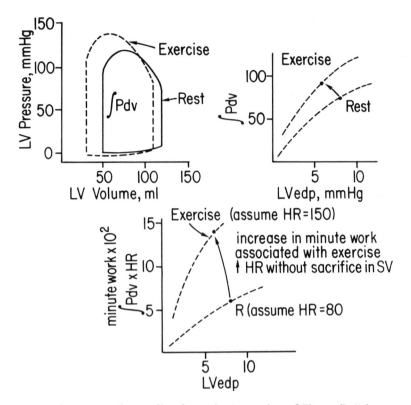

FIGURE 7–2 Exercise cardiac dynamics (extension of Figure 7–1) in terms of the Frank–Starling–Sarnoff relationship. In the upper left figure rest and upright exercise PV loops are shown from which stroke work (∫ Pdv) is obtained. Plotting these against LV end-diastolic pressure (edp) in the upper right figure shows the positive inotropic effect of exercise; that is, exercise point on a curve above and leftward of the control curve. However, because this does not take heart rate change during exercise into account, in the bottom figure minute ventricular work (stroke work × heart rate) is plotted on the ordinate to emphasize how positive inotropy allows the heart to function as a constant stroke pump where rate is the dominant determinant of output.

block sympathetic β-receptors, respectively? What cardiac output responses are possible in such circumstances?

Exercise, expecially repetitive isotonic exercise (such as running or swimming) where large muscle masses are involved, is an effective way significantly and independently to enhance venous return to the heart. The normal heart and especially the conditioned heart will pump out what it gets, utilizing the length–tension relationship in the absence of all else. In addition, remember that in denervating the greyhound heart, nothing was done to the adrenal medulla; thus, the heart rate and contractility did increase albeit submaximally in response to increased circulating epinephrine. Patients on reserpine and propranolol get by, but they are not prone to vigorous activity. Besides, there are the previously discussed compensatory mechanisms nature provided: O_2 delivery exceeding need by a comfortable margin, which provides a limited but readily available store of oxygen; the remarkable qualities of the oxygen-carrying respiratory pigment, hemoglobin; and finally, a mechanism for controlling distribution of cardiac output (Chapter 12).

8

THE ARTERIAL SYSTEM

In December I caused a mare to be tied down alive on her back; she was
14 hands high, and about 14 years of age, had a fistula on her withers,
was neither very lean nor yet lusty: having laid open the left crural artery
about 3 inches from her belly, I inserted into it a brass pipe whose bore
was $1/6$ of an inch in diameter; and to that, by means of another brass
pipe which was fitly adated to it, I fixed a glass tube, of nearly the same
diameter, which was 9 feet in length: then untying the ligature on the
artery, the blood rose in the tube 8 feet 3 inches perpendicular above the
level of the left ventricle of the heart: but it did not attain to its full height
at once; it rushed up about half way in an instant, and afterwards gradually at each pulse, 12, 8, 6, 4, 2 and sometimes 1 inch: when it was at its
full height, it would rise and fall at and after each pulse 2, 3, or 4 inches
. . .

STEPHEN HALES.
*Statical Essays: An Account of Some Hydraulic and Hydrostatical Experiments
made on the Blood and Blood Vessels of Animals.*
London, 1733.

It requires energy to move fluid through a tube system and the energy is in both potential (pressure) and kinetic (flow velocity) form.
The heart is able to add energy to blood because of the arrangement
of valves and the discontinuous (cyclic) nature of pumping which
allows ventricular filling to occur at low energy expenditure while
heart muscle rests. When heart muscle contracts, it generates tension—in effect squeezes—raising the pressure of the incompressible
fluid contents trapped in its cavity. How high the pressure will rise
before the exit valve opens and pressure is translated to fluid movement (ejection) depends on the pressure in the arterial outflow vessel
at the time (i.e., at the end of diastole). This raises a very important
question: What determines the pressure in arteries?

The arterial blood pressure varies tremendously from species to
species, from individual to individual within a species, and from time
to time in a given individual. For example, consider the differences
among the average resting arterial pressure of the frog (30/20), pi-
geon (180/130), man (120/80), and giraffe (250/180). Stephen Hales'
mare had a mean arterial pressure of about 190 mm Hg, undoubtedly

an unphysiologic value. Why does there seem to be so much quantitative variety in accomplishing perfusion?

Nature, having had billions of years to work its wonders, you can bet with some confidence that there is a good reason behind most biologic phenomena. You know that nature abhors vacuums; it also abhors wasting valuable biologic energy. The question might then be raised: Why, if it is possible for some species to survive with so little pressure, do others have to generate so much? The cardiac energy expenditure to develop blood pressure far exceeds that required to add kinetic energy to the blood; therefore, it is reasonable to expect that nature would avoid the requirement for more pressure than was biologically necessary.

What determines whether pressure will be high or low for any given blood flow? A more fundamental question would be: What is responsible for pressure, period?

DISTENSIBILITY AND STATIC
VERSUS DYNAMIC VOLUMES AND PRESSURES

The heart chambers and all the blood vessels in the body taken together have a maximum capacity that may be as much as twice the actual blood volume. It is literally possible to bleed to death within one's own vascular space (i.e., without a drop of blood leaving the circulation). Ordinarily, only a part of the vascular capacity is used at any given moment; this applies particularly to capillary and venous beds. The reason this is brought up here is because the main determinants of pressure are the distensibility characteristic of the vascular compartment and the volume of blood contained therein. This applies to the whole system or any part of it and to dynamic as well as static conditions.

Distensibility, the ratio of volume to pressure change, of heart chambers and especially blood vessels is a complex matter, for vascular wall is made up of varying quantities of different tissues, each with its own characteristic stress–strain (or length–tension) relationship. Smooth muscle in vascular wall adds another dimension of complexity because its stress–strain relationship varies as a function of the state of its contraction. Another complexity, especially in aorta and large arteries of man, is that distensibility is markedly affected by atherosclerosis, so-called hardening of the arteries, so common with aging. In general, however, distensibility of most vessels is reasonably linear over a narrow physiologic range, especially when there is only resting smooth muscle tone. Beyond the physiologic range, especially in arteries, distensibility diminishes strikingly because it is then primarily determined by the tough (i.e., stiff), fibrous adventitia. The distensibility of veins is orders-of-magnitude greater than of arteries. This, plus the fact that at each level veins are roughly twice the diameter of corresponding arteries, explains why most of the blood in the vascular space is in the veins (cross-sectional area 4X). Actually, this difference in blood distribution between arteries and veins is magnified further when the heart beat stops.

It is a simple experiment to stop the heart beat temporarily (such as by strong vagal stimulation) while measuring arterial and venous blood pressure. What would be observed is that arterial pressure falls rapidly and venous pressure rises slowly until they both reach the same value. This value is referred to as mean circulatory filling pressure, is about 7 mm Hg in the anesthetized dog and represents the static volume/pressure relation free of external energy input. The observed pressure changes occur because blood continues to leave the arterial system and capillaries and drains into the venous system until the energy producing this transfer is dissipated. At this uniform pressure, almost all the blood volume would be in veins. On restarting the heart (assume no reflexes occurred in the meantime) the arterial pressure would not reach its original level until the distribution of blood had been restored to its dynamic state. The effect of the heart beat, therefore, is to keep a certain volume of blood on the arterial side that under static conditions would be on the venous side. This dynamic redistribution results from the high-outflow resistance of the arterial system afforded by the muscular arterioles and precapillary sphincters into which the heart pumps blood. This shifted extra volume pumped into the relatively indistensible aorta and large arterial vessel produces the high arterial pressures characteristic of all birds and mammals. Thus, as shown in Figure 8–1, mean arterial pressure in a given species or individual is determined by the ratio of inflow rate (cardiac output) to arterial outflow conductance. (Phasic changes in blood pressure involve the distensibility of arterial vessels, the heart rate, and time course of ejection as well.) A simple common analog of this system is the dust-collecting canvas or paper bag of an upright floor vacuum cleaner. Such bags become pressurized when the

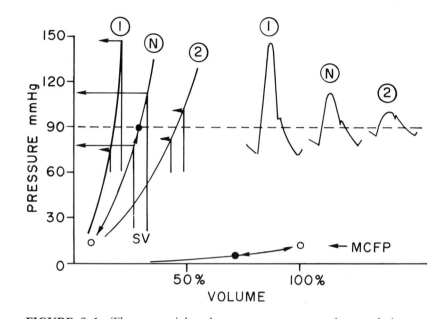

FIGURE 8-1 Three arterial and a venous pressure–volume relations to illustrate their role in determining mean and phasic arterial pressures. Curve N shows normal, curve 1 diminished and curve 2 increased arterial distensibility or compliance. The closed circles on curve N and venous curve at bottom. represent pressure–volume points when the heart is beating showing that of total systemic blood volume (abscissa) roughly 70% is in the veins and capillaries and 25% in the arteries. If the heart were stopped, arterial pressure and volume would fall along arterial distensibility curve N and venous pressure rise along its PV curve until both pressures equalized at the open circles, a value known as the mean circulatory filling pressure (MCFP) when virtually all the blood would be in the veins. Thus the heart beat produces dynamic redistribution of static volumes shifting a portion from venous to arterial side. The right ventricle is interposed between these vascular volumes in mammalian circulations and it plays a role in redistribution. The different distensibility curves show how different redistribution volumes (less for stiff and more for compliant) would be required to produce a given mean arterial pressure and how systolic, diastolic and pulse pressure (arrows pointing leftward) would differ when the same stroke volume (SV) is injected into each system (pressure pulses on right).

machine is turned on because the fan pumps air into the bag faster than it can leak out until the steady state pressure and volume are reached. The greater this input–output discrepancy, the higher the steady-state pressure. (The analogy is limited, however, because such bags have substantially different distensibility characteristics.)

THE WINDKESSEL FUNCTION

Two important benefits accrue from this particular arrangement. First, the highly elastic aorta and large arteries combine with the high-outflow resistance to convert intermittent flow (the stroke volume) into nearly steady flow at the capillary level. What happens is that a certain portion of the stroke volume is absorbed into distending the vessel walls during ejection and is therefore subtracted from systolic flow. During diastole this stored volume with its accompanying potential energy (i.e., stretched elastic fibers) is available to augment diastolic pressure and flow out of the system. This temporary storage property of the aorta and large arterial vessels referred to as the windkessel (compression chamber) function is illustrated in Figure 8–2. The reader is reminded that some lower vertebrates (elasmobranchs, fish) have a separate (valved) chamber interposed between the ventricle and aorta, the bulbus cordis or arteriosus, that is highly elastic and may have cardiac muscle too, that serves a similar depulsating function.

CONTROL OF BLOOD PRESSURE AND FLOW DISTRIBUTION

Early in this survey it was pointed out that not only did the metabolic activity and, therefore, the oxygen requirement of the various tissues differ, they were variable within a given tissue from time to time. For skeletal muscle, the range of oxygen consumption can be as much as 50-fold. How is this vast range of blood flow requirements among tissues met? The mechanism that nature devised for meeting these is basically the same one that man rediscovered when electricity was discovered and put to use: parallel circuits and ohmic resistance.

In parallel means the arrangement wherein branches to each organ come directly off the main line, which has the effect of exposing each and every organ to common aortic blood pressure. This type of system will function properly when the capacity of the energy source to generate pressure (or voltage in the case of electricity) exceeds that which can be dissipated as flow energy in the branches when outflow resistance is at a minimum. (What happens when you short out an electric outlet? The average American home has virtually unlimited electric power for ordinary use, but circuits are fused to keep maximum current flow within the limits of the capacity of wiring to con-

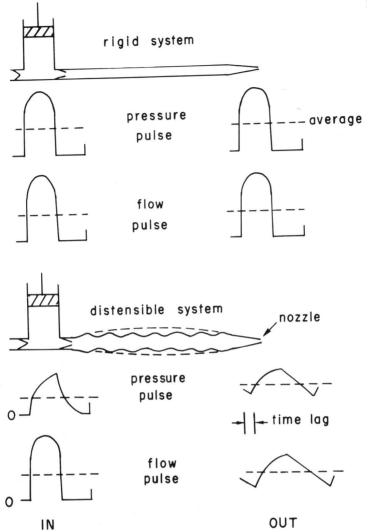

FIGURE 8–2 The windkessel (compression chamber) effect. In the rigid system depicted above intermittent strokes of the pump on the left injects a volume into the tube within a certain time and raises the pressure and velocity of the liquid in a pulsatile way (pressure and flow pulse IN). At the restricted nozzle end of the tube on the right the pressure and flow pulses OUT will occur virtually simultaneously if the medium is an incompressible liquid. Thus intermittent (interrupted) outflow will occur. In the distensible tube system below, the same input volume pulse will produce a different pressure pulse (lower peak, longer time to peak and delayed return to zero pressure between cycles). The output flow pulse is quite different in that it is less intermittent and the pulse delayed slightly. The latter is due to effect of elasticity on pulse wave transmission and the former to the fact that the combination of the high outflow resistance (the nozzle) and the distensible tube walls will cause some of the inflow stroke volume to distend the tube rather than flow out. The energy stored in the elastic walls is then dissipated after the inflow cycle ceases as continued flow out of the nozzle.

duct it without overheating.) In the circulation, the number of potential circuits exceeds the capacity of the unconditioned pump when the former are all open maximally simultaneously. In the latter circumstances, pressure falls to low levels and the animal is said to be in shock (Chapter 15).

Arterial beds connected in parallel represent pathways competing for blood flow to the extent that the amount available for distribution is not infinite. One of the more remarkable aspects of the circulatory system is the manner in which blood flow distribution is regulated to suit demand considering the variability of the latter. It is a matter of control of vascular resistance.

VASCULAR RESISTANCE OR CONDUCTANCE

Resistance (R) may be defined as the property of a tube or blood vessel to impede the flow of fluid within it. In this sense it is analogous to the use of the term in electricity where current flow in a conductor rather than fluid flow is considered. Some prefer to use the reciprocal term conductance (G), the property of conductivity, and there is some advantage to being able to think in direct rather than inverse terms, especially in parallel circuits.

$$R = \frac{1}{G}.$$

If you were a highway, water, sewer, or electrical power engineer and you were asked to design a system for a city, one of the first things you would want to know is the peak, as well as average, demand that would be placed on the system. Your ultimate design would take into account both requirements and probably include a safety factor as well. So it is with nature and blood vessels. The vascularity (capillary density) of each tissue is such that maximum rather than average or resting needs can be met. This means that to the extent there is less than maximum activity and flow, there is excess vascularity. In a sleeping heavyweight weightlifter, this excess vascularity in skeletal muscle is enormous. Thus, there has to be a mechanism that permits conductance to be adjusted directly proportional to demand in each tissue and the sum of all these must be within the energy output capacity of the heart.

In electricity, as you know, the resistance (R) of a conductor is the ratio of voltage drop between two points (ΔE) and the current flow (I)

$$R \text{ (ohms)} = \frac{\Delta E}{I}.$$

The value of electric resistance varies as a function of the material from which the conductor is made, its size or gauge, and temperature. The concept of hydrodynamic resistance actually was developed in 1840 before George Ohm conceived that of ohmic resistance by a French physician, Jean-Leonard-Marie Poiseuille, who carefully studied the factors that determined the flow of water in fine glass tubes. He was really interested in blood flow in blood vessels but settled for water in glass tubes because he soon found blood and blood vessels too difficult to work with. The result of Poiseuille's experiments led to the empirical formulation of the following equation describing the determinants of fluid flow

$$\dot{Q} = \frac{\Delta P \, \pi r^4}{8 \, L \eta}$$

where $\dot{Q}$ = flow rate, ΔP = pressure gradient, drop or difference across tube, r = radius of tube, L = length of tube, η = viscosity of fluid.

What Poiseuille discovered was that for a given glass tube, the flow of water was directly proportional to the pressure drop. The proportionality constant, R, describing the relationship of pressure gradient to flow is

$$R = \frac{\Delta P}{\dot{Q}} = \frac{8 \, L \eta}{\pi \, r^4}$$

and the analogy to ohmic resistance becomes obvious. Assuming for the moment that viscosity and tube length are also constant and collecting all the constant terms together as K, one gets

$$R = \frac{K}{r^4} = \frac{\Delta P}{\dot{Q}} \text{ and } G = \frac{r^4}{K} = \frac{\dot{Q}}{\Delta P}.$$

(In Poiseuille's experiments even r was constant for a given tube.) This simplifed equation shows that the proportionality constant that we call resistance (R) is inversely and conductance, G, directly proportional to the radius of the tube raised to the fourth power (Figure

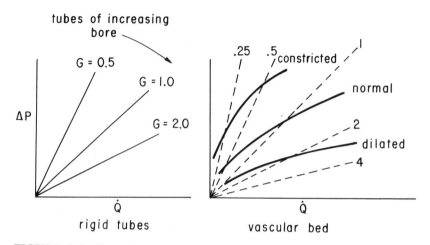

FIGURE 8–3 Vascular conductance, G, or its reciprocal, resistance. In the lefthand panel linear flow-pressure gradient relations of tubes of different bore show how calculated indices $G = \dot{Q}/\Delta P$ and $R = \Delta P/\dot{Q}$ are accurate descriptors of tube flow conductive or resistance properties. In the right panel a single vascular bed under three states of vasomotor activity have the same general relationship as tubes of different bore on the left but that in none of the individual curves is it possible to describe the flow–pressure gradient relation by a single conductance or resistance value because of nonlinearity.

8–3). This means that if r is variable, small changes in it would result in large changes in resistance. What Poiseuille obviously found during his experiments was that very small differences in tube bore made large differences in flow, all other things being equal.

Biologic vascular systems are a lot more complicated than described by $R = \Delta P/\dot{Q}$, but as a first-order approximation and especially as a conceptual tool, it has great value. The important thing is that knowledge of readily measurable physiologic variables, pressure gradient and flow, provides significant insight into the flow conducting or resisting properties of the inaccessible blood vessels, especially in terms of their bore and changes therein.

We can now return to the question posed earlier concerning what determines arterial blood pressure (BP) by invoking the resistance concept substituting cardiac output for $\dot{Q}$ and making the acceptable assumption that the value for BP represents the total pressure drop across the systemic circulation (i.e., assume right atrial pressure is zero).

$$BP = CO \times R \text{ or } BP = \frac{CO}{G}.$$

(Remember $R = K/r^4$.) This indicates that BP is maintained by the ratio of CO to the bore of vessels somewhere in the atrial system. For example, if vessels became smaller (decrease in r), R would increase by the fourth power; and if CO remained the same, BP would also rise by the same amount.

PRESSURE GRADIENTS IN THE SYSTEMIC CIRCULATION (FIGURE 8-4)

Since the capillary pressure in man must be 25–30 mm Hg and the right atrial pressure is about zero, approximately 25–30% of pressure energy generated by the heart is expended in returning blood to the heart from the capillaries, and this pressure drop is more or less evenly distributed along the entire venous path. The distribution of pressure drop in the arterial system is dramatically different. There is a small (10–15%) gradual loss of pressure between the aortic root and the small distal arteries (of perhaps 0.5–1.0 mm diameter), but from that point to the arterial end of the capillaries, the pressure drops precipitously by the remaining 55–65% unaccounted previously to the level of capillary pressure. The vessels over which this major drop occurs are characterized by abundant smooth muscle, rich sympathetic innervation, and are called arterioles. These vessels together with the precapillary sphincters, therefore, represent the loci of major resistance to egress of blood from the arterial system and account for most of the R of $BP = CO \times R$. It is the control of the bore of these vessels that determines the distribution of blood flow to tissues and to capillaries. This is precisely analogous to how current flow in the electric wiring in a home or hospital is determined by the electric resistance (or conductance) of each light, appliance or machine when it is switched on given an adequate voltage source. Remember that in parallel circuits the total conductance of a system is the sum of all the individual conductances:

$$G \text{ (total)} = g_1 + g_2 + g_3 \cdots + g_n.$$

(In series circuits the total resistance is the sum of the individual resistances: $R \text{ (total)} = R_1 + R_2 + R_3 \cdots + R_n$.) Thus, because BP = CO/G, it should be apparent why, when all the arterioles and

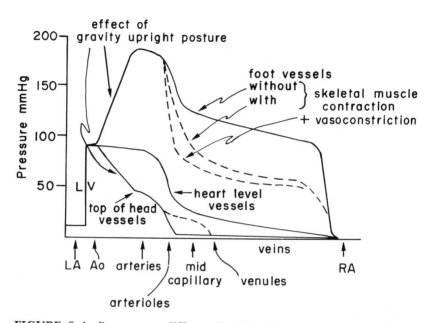

FIGURE 8–4 Pressures at different levels in the systemic circulation and the effect of gravity in the erect posture. Left ventricular contraction at the left raises the pressure energy of the blood from the low level in the left atrium to about 90 mm Hg in the aorta. In heart-level vessels (i.e., no gravitational effect) this pressure is progressively dissipated as the pressure gradient producing flow. However, the major drop is across the arterioles because it is the flow conductive properties of these vessels that causes the arterial pressure to be high and the capillary pressure to be regulated at a level (25–30 mm Hg) near that of plasma osmotic pressure. The upper and lower curves illustrate the substantial effect of gravity on these pressures in upright man. Also shown (dotted lines) are beneficial effects such as the skeletal muscle pump (Chapter 10), arterial vasoconstriction and venous collapse above heart level (lower dotted line) on these gravitational distortions, particularly the effect of the skeletal muscle pump in lowering high venous pressure in the legs.

sphincters are paralyzed (maximum G), BP may fall even though CO is significantly increased. Muscular effort represents a circumstance where the conductance of vessels supplying contracting muscle increases. If there are enough of these, G (total) may be markedly increased; despite this, BP during exercise even in patients with heart disease usually is increased. This obviously means that the increase in CO more than compensates for the increase in vascular conductance.

We suggested earlier that nature would be loathe to waste precious biologic energy. Why then is BP in certain species maintained so much higher than that necessary to maintain capillary pressure at 25–30 mm Hg? This question defies a unified explanation considering the extraordinary variability in BP among the species with no discernible pattern, but certain situations do lend themselves to reasonable explanation.

EFFECT OF GRAVITY ON ARTERIAL PRESSURE

Whatever the BP is in the root of the aorta, relatively it is 1 mm Hg less for each 1.36 cm of vertical distance above the heart level and the same amount more below heart level. This effect is mediated by gravity acting on the uninterrupted fluid column. In upright man, therefore, arterial pressure at the top of the head is 40 mm Hg or so less than at heart level on this account. This pressure loss in the giraffe may be as much as 200 mm Hg! Thus, because brain perfusion cannot be sacrificed under any circumstances, heart-level BP must be high enough to overcome the gravitational effect and still have some margin of safety. It should be obvious that the requirement to perfuse the brain, the vertical distance above the heart which is so substantial, imposes in such animals the opposite problem of high pressure in vessels below heart level. By and large, nature seems to have succeeded in overcoming this problem permitting man to be upright and the giraffe to eat the leaves of trees, but there is a not uncommon clinical condition called orthostatic hypotension which is characterized by fainting or tendency thereto during erect posture. Fighter pilots during World War II also discovered that nature had not equipped them to prevent black-out during the augmentation of strong positive gravitational force that accompany pulling out of a dive or banking sharply at high speed.

The energy cost to the heart of generating high arterial blood pressure is a matter of survival for the giraffe and is, therefore, well worth paying. The rationale for high-blood pressure in other species not having to cope with gravitational considerations, such as birds and snakes, remains enigmatic.

To summarize, arterial blood pressure is determined by the ratio of cardiac output to the total conductance of the vascular system. Total conductance is determined by the sum of all individual conductances (i.e., parallel paths). The latter, in turn, is determined by the sum of all resistances in series in each individual branch. The balance of this ratio (CO/G) provides for the more or less characteristic value for BP in each species. In species with low BP, the ratio favors conductance whereas in those with high pressure it favors flow (active species). The regulated variable of the trio is BP; thus, changes in total conductance resulting from changes in individual conductances must be accompanied by proportional changes in CO for BP to remain steady. The value of and changes in individual conductances result mainly from the state of contraction of vascular smooth muscle in the walls of arterioles and precapillary sphincters. Such vasomotor tone changes not only contribute to the maintenance of BP, they provide a mechanism to regulate capillary hydrostatic pressure to maintain tissue water homeostasis.

PRESSURE TRANSMISSION IN THE ARTERIAL SYSTEM

The cyclic ejection of the stroke volume into the aortic root produces repeating pulses of time varying pressure. The pressure contour depends on factors such as frequency, volume and rate of ejection, the pressure in the aortic root at the time ejection commences, the status of peripheral resistance, and the lumped elasticity or distensibility of the aorta and major arterial branches. In a rigid tube system, the transmission of the pulse and of incompressible fluid virtually coincides. In other words, fluid moves out the other end with negligible phase lag in the rate of volume and pressure that is being put in. In a distensible system, things are more complex, especially when distensibility itself is not constant with respect to volume and elasticity is accompanied by viscosity. In this setting not only does the transmission of the pressure wave (5×10^2 cm/sec) markedly precede the flow wave (30 cm/sec), both are altered considerably during the process of transmission such that what comes out the other end is substantially different than what is put in. First of all, there is transmission delay of the pressure wave. However, this delay is not great because pulse wave transmission is rapid (5 m/sec) compared to the length of the system. Second, velocity of transmission seems to vary as a function of pressure; that is, a given pressure increment is transmitted faster when the pressure is high than when the level is low. This may be a mechanism for the observation that the peak tends to catch up or move forward with respect to the onset and tail of the pressure pulse. Another explanation that has been offered is that the

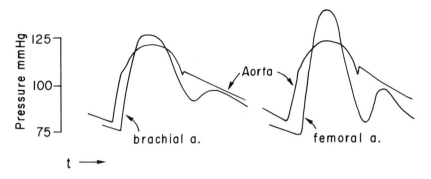

FIGURE 8–5 Changes in aortic pressure pulse associated with transmission to peripheral (brachial and femoral) arteries. Note loss of sharp transients such as anacrotic shoulder on upstroke and incisura (closure of aortic valve) on downstroke due to damping. Most striking effects include appearance of secondary (dicrotic) trough and wave, enhancement of peak systolic pressure and steepening of upstroke, effects due, at least in part, to wave reflection.

rate of pressure change itself is a determinant of transmission velocity, a steeper rate of change, such as occurs in the early part of the pressure pulse being transmitted faster. The high arteriolar resistance at the end of the system also is thought to contribute to distortion of the pulse wave during transmission. The notion is that a secondary or reflected wave is set up in the periphery that bounces back along the system. This wave too is damped during its transmission so that it fails to reach the central pulse.

Whatever the mechanisms, the pressure pulse in the aortic root is significantly altered during its transmission to peripheral vessels. As shown in Figure 8–5, the characteristic features of this alteration are that the peak becomes sharper, systolic pressure increases in absolute magnitude (by as much as 20–30 mm Hg), high-frequency transients are damped out so that the wave becomes smoothed out, and a second positive wave appears during early diastole (the dicrotic wave). These effects are more exaggerated the farther out the system one goes up to a point; beyond that, progressive branching and narrowing increases damping which flattens pressure fluctuation.

ANATOMIC–PHYSIOLOGIC ASPECTS OF BRANCHING

The cross-sectional area of the vascular system increases progressively from the aortic root to the capillaries because of branching. One might well ask why resistance is localized to arterioles and precapillary sphincters despite the ever-widening stream? The answer has to do, at least in part, with the physical consequences of the anatomy of branching.

According to the Poiseuille relationship, the cross-sectional area of equal-sized offspring branches must be $\sqrt{n}$ times that of the parent vessel (n being the number of branches) if resistance is to remain unchanged. For example, for four branches the summed cross section must be double that of the parent, for nine branches, three times, etc. Obviously resistance will increase or decrease to the extent this relationship either is not met or is exceeded (i.e., $< \sqrt{n}$ or $> \sqrt{n}$). This means that a physical mechanism exists for resistance to increase with branching even though summed cross section is increasing as long as the latter is less than $\sqrt{n}$. Similarly, resistance can be decreased by an arrangement whereby the summed cross section of branches exceeds $\sqrt{n}$. Recruitment, the opening of previously closed branches, therefore, represents an ingeniously simple way for getting more blood to a tissue with minimal energy expenditure. It is probable that nature uses this principle to achieve high systemic arteriolar resistance and low capillary resistance. In the lung airways and vasculature, this principle affords a low resistance at all levels.

AUTOREGULATION

Autoregulation is the term given to an experimental phenomenon wherein flow to an organ after an initial change returns to the control or constant level despite a rather wide range of perfusion pressure gradient. First demonstrated in the kidney, it has since been found to occur in the brain, heart, and resting skeletal muscle. The magnitude of this effect is variable but consider the physiologic significance of the phenomenon: Organs/tissues exhibiting it resist being overperfused (wasted flow) or underperfused (rendered ischemic) relative to their oxygen needs by automatic quantitatively appropriate adjustments of vasomotor tone such that vascular conductance decreases as perfusion pressure gradient (ΔP) is increased or increases as ΔP is diminished. That this mechanism functions in real life is demonstrated by observations of normal organ blood flow in human hypertension. What local mechanism accounts for this interesting phenomenon remains unproved, but perhaps the two most durable hypotheses are the myogenic and metabolic theories. The first postulates that an inherent property of vascular smooth muscle is one wherein an imposed stretching force is counteracted by contraction whereas diminished force the opposite (i.e., relaxation). How this is mediated has yet to be elucidated. In the second, tissue metabolism at a given level results in the presence (elaboration) of a certain amount of some vasodilator substance (e.g., P_{O_2}, P_{CO_2}, pH, adenosine); tendency to hyperperfusion is resisted by vasoconstriction because incremental washout lowers local concentration of the substance. Contrarily, hypoperfusion tendency is resisted by buildup of the substance locally leading to vasodilation.

9
CAPILLARY CIRCULATION

Harvey correctly deduced that blood distributed by arteries returned to the heart via veins, but he was rather vague about the interconnection. He used descriptions such as: "the obscure porosities of the lungs and the minute inosculations of vessels," blood having to "percolate the parenchyma of the lungs" and "· · · or pores in the flesh and solid parts generally that are permeable to the blood." Quite clearly he was close to the truth a quarter century before capillaries were visualized through microscopes by Malpighi and van Leeuwenhoek. The latter wrote (1708)

> These three distinct vessels with their somewhat circular course, in which the circulation took place, where so small that a grain of sand could have covered them." "If now we see clearly with our eyes that the passing of the blood from the arteries into the veins, in the tadpoles, only takes place in such blood vessels as are so thin that only one corpuscle can be driven through at one time, we may conclude that the same thing takes place in the same way in our bodies as well as in that of all animals.

Malpighi's description (1661)

> I had believed that this body of the blood breaks into the empty space, and is collected again by a gaping vessel and by structure of the walls ... But the dried lung of the frog made my belief dubious. This lung had, by chance, preserved the redness of the blood in the smallest vessels, where by means of a more perfect lens, no more met the eye but vessels mingled annularly. And, so great is the divarification of these vessels as they go out, here from a vein, there from an artery, that order is no longer preserved, but a network appears made up of the prolongation of both vessels. . . . it was clear to sense that the blood flows away through the tortuous vessels, that it is not poured into spaces but always works through tubules and is dispersed by the multiplex winding of the vessels.

It was indicated in Chapter 2 that the function of the circulation is served at the level of the capillary–interstitial fluid interface because this is where the process of diffusion exchange takes place that maintains a physiologic cellular environment with respect to a number and variety of substances that either are needed or produced by functioning cells. Oxygen supply (and CO_2 removal) was identified as the index parameter since the homeostatic mechanisms seem to be geared to this end. Cell hydration would easily qualify for the position of a close second. As with all substances, the amount of water in a given tissue is the steady-state balance between the amount supplied to and removed from the interstitial fluid. It is appropriate now to consider the forces that govern water distribution.

CAPILLARY FLUID DYNAMICS

Capillary endothelium can be thought of as a highly leaky membrane that offers no impediment to free diffusion of water and small solute particles, such as ions as well as of gases. Indeed, such diffusion exchange between capillary bed and cell water is so free that injected isotopically labeled water or potassium reaches equilibrium with tissue water or potassium during a single circulatatory pass. The reason for this is that the capillary surface area is very large and the diffusion distance very short. Variations in capillary endothelial morphology and permeability have a greater bearing on whether larger molecules are able to pass through. The existence, magnitude, and direction of concentration gradients for water among plasma, interstitial fluid, and cell water are variable from moment to moment, but in all likelihood this is not a major exchange factor.

While diffusion is responsible for free exchange of water among the three compartments, it does not account for the net balance of fluid distribution in tissues. This is governed by other forces.

Osmotic Pressure of Plasma

Osmosis is the force resulting from differences in solute concentration of solutions separated by a membrane having the special property of allowing solvent to pass through either exclusively or at least far more easily than solute (semipermeable). Osmotic pressure is merely a convenient way to express the magnitude of this force. Osmotic pressure is directly related to the total number of particles in solution, and in situations where the solutions on either side of a membrane have different concentrations of the same or different solutes, it is the difference in particle concentration that determines osmotic pressure. The species or size of particle is not what is important. The total osmotic pressure of plasma is very high, almost 8 atmospheres! The particles responsible for this huge pressure are primarily ions: Na^+, Cl^-, HCO_3^-, Ca^{++}, K^+, $PO_4\equiv$, etc. A much smaller amount is due to substances such as glucose, urea, creatinine, etc., and a miniscule remainder due to the plasma proteins, albumin, and globulins. In the body, however, the latter, especially albumin, dominate the picture because all the others are so small and diffusible that they are distributed across the capillary membrane in virtually identical concentration; thus, exerting no differential osmotic force. The effective or so-called colloid osmotic pressure of plasma (π pl), therefore, is a mere approximately 25–30 mm Hg in man and most mammals, 10–15 in birds, 7–10 in amphibia, and 4–5 in fishes. Human plasma protein concentration accounting for this osmotic (or oncotic) pressure is approximately 7 g%, slightly over half albumin. Albumin molecules account for all but a small fraction of protein osmotic pressure, however, because of the marked differences in molecular size (i.e., approximately 70,000 for albumin versus few to several 100,000s mw for globulins).

Capillary Hydrostatic (Filtration) Pressure and Its Determinants

Plasma colloid osmotic pressure (PCOP) may be small in magnitude but it is extremely important in circulatory homeostasis. Unopposed, the force would result in water being absorbed from the interstitial fluid space and, ultimately, from cells into the circulation. Thus, one of the fundamental requirements of the cardiovascular system is to establish and critically regulate a pressure of equal magnitude but opposite in direction to offset the cell-dehydrating force of PCOP. This means that whatever arterial pressure is, 25–30 mm Hg of it must be available at the capillary level in most tissues most of the time for this purpose.

Since capillary hydrostatic presure (Pc) is regulated to balance PCOP, it is important to consider its determinants. In most species, but especially in mammals, birds, and snakes, arterial blood pressure is substantially higher than optimal capillary hydrostatic pressure. Arteriolar constrictor tone provides a mechanism for reducing high-arterial pressure, but at the same time this mechanism is what makes arterial pressure high. Because there is another factor involved in determining blood pressure independent of arteriolar tone (i.e., cardiac output), it turns out that both blood pressure and arteriolar tone are determinants of capillary pressure.

Another determinant of capillary hydrostatic pressure is the level of venous pressure. Excluding gravitational effects, venous pressure is significantly lower than capillary hydrostatic pressure, posing no impediment to capillary drainage downstream. If venous pressure is elevated for any reason, Pc tends to rise, all other things remaining equal. Dependency (i.e., below heart level) is a physiologic and congestive heart failure or venous disease (such as varicose veins) pathologic conditions wherein venous pressure is elevated. Such conditions are usually attended by some degree of excessive tissue fluid accumulation (edema) due to concomitant elevation of capillary hydrostatic pressure.

Capillary hydrostatic pressure also varies as a function of venous smooth muscle (so-called venomotor) tone, especially of the small veins just downstream from the capillary. Constriction of such muscles (venoconstriction), all other factors remaining unchanged, results in elevation of capillary pressure; relaxation the opposite. Such effects alter the ease of egress of blood from the capillary network and raise or lower Pc. This may be one of the mechanisms by which substances such as histamine produce tissue edema.

Finally, two other general factors may influence capillary pressure: total blood volume and cardiac output. All other things remaining equal, the higher these are the higher arterial and venous pressures would tend to be and capillary pressure accordingly. Such changes do occur in acute renal diseases or inadvertent iatrogenic (physician caused) fluid replacement volume overload. The opposite occurs in volume depletion states such as dehydration (e.g., as in cholera) or blood loss.

Quite obviously, regulation of capillary hydrostatic pressure is a very complex phenomenon considering the number of variables involved. It would be a mistake to think that all these factors are finely adjusted on a moment-to-moment basis to maintain optimal tissue fluid balance. Each of these variables is important to other physiologic phenomena and the body economy assigns them different priority depending on the particular circumstance. For example, in acute hemorrhagic shock, blood pressure is low despite maximal arteriolar and venular constriction. Low Pc in this setting allows interstitial fluid resorption, an effect which helps compensate for volume depletion and to maintain cardiac output.

No discussion of capillary fluid dynamics would be complete without mentioning two other variables: tissue (or interstitial fluid) pressure and tissue fluid osmotic pressure.

Tissue Pressure

Tissue pressure is the hydrostatic pressure of the interstitial fluid space. It is somewhat variable from tissue to tissue and except inside closed rigid spaces, such as in the skull, spinal canal, and bone marrow, it is variable from time to time. Mainly it reflects the relationship between tissue (including cells) volume and the distensibility characteristics (volume–pressure relationship) of that tissue. Under ordinary circumstances, this relationship is such that interstitial fluid pressure (Pi.f.) is maintained at low levels, 0–2 mm Hg. There are even claims that it is negative (i.e., subatmospheric). The distensibility of a tissue or organ has to do with its structure and composition, bone and endocrine glands being examples at opposite ends of the spectrum. The capsules of organs such as kidney, liver, and spleen confer one kind of distensibility and the enclosure of the brain in the skull another. Very small volume changes of the skull contents are accompanied by marked pressure rise, whereas the spleen can swell to many times its original volume with modest pressure increment, especially if it occurs gradually. Similarly, human lower extremity subcutaneous soft tissue accomodates edema fluid readily, whereas the giraffe is protected from this by tough, unyielding hide. Thus, Pi.f. ordinarily represents only a small opposing force to capillary filtration, but under certain circumstances it may become limiting.

Interstitial Fluid Osmotic Pressure

Interstitial fluid osmotic pressure (Π.i.f.) is that owing to the presence of small amounts of plasma proteins that escape from capillaries. Obviously its magnitude is accordingly small, approximately 1–3 mm Hg. These proteins eventually exit through lymphatics to reenter the circulation. In organs or tissues where large amounts of proteins are produced, such as the liver, on the other hand, Π.i.f. is not negligible. Since capillary/sinusoidal pressure in the liver is quite low because of the portal circulation, the balance of forces is different than in most other tissues.

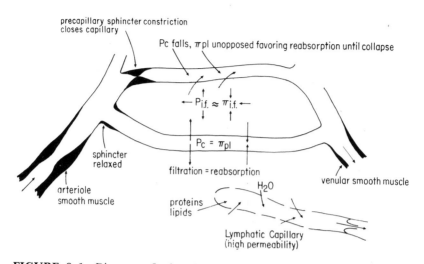

precapillary sphincter constriction
closes capillary

Pc falls, πpl unopposed favoring reabsorption until collapse

$\leftarrow P_{i.f.} \approx \pi_{i.f.} \leftarrow$

$P_c = \pi_{pl}$

sphincter
relaxed

filtration = reabsorption

arteriole
smooth muscle

H_2O

venular smooth muscle

proteins
lipids

Lymphatic Capillary
(high permeability)

FIGURE 9-1 Diagram of microcirculation showing blood entering via arteriole on left and leaving via venule and lymphatic vessel (as lymph) on right. Major bidirectional fluid exchange across capillary membrane is by diffusion but hydrodynamic component due to Starling–Landis forces is depicted: P_c = capillary hydrostatic (filtration), πpl = plasma osmotic (reabsorption), Pi.f. = interstitial fluid hydrostatic (reabsorption), πi.f. interstitial fluid osmotic (filtration) pressures. In certain tissues high permeability of lymphatic capillary endothelium provides avenues for absorption of macromolecules into the circulation.

STARLING HYPOTHESIS

Ernest Starling first proposed a hypothesis describing the balance of all the above forces operating at the level of the capillaries to maintain tissue water balance. This Law of the Capillaries has been as enduring as his Law of the Heart. Eugene Landis contributed so much in establishing its validity that it is now known as the Starling–Landis hypothesis of capillary fluid dynamics. It can be stated in its simplest form as an equation

$$FM = \frac{k[(Pc + II.i.f.)}{\text{filtration}} - \frac{(Pi.f. + IIpl.)]}{\text{reabsorption}}.$$

In the situation where there is no *net* fluid movement (FM) into or out of the capillary (obviously great amounts are passing in both directions because of diffusion exchange), FM = 0 and the sums of the items in parentheses are equal in magnitude but opposite in sign, filtration versus reabsorption. This is depicted in Figure 9–1.

10

VENOUS AND LYMPHATIC SYSTEMS

The effect of this arrangement (of venous valves) plainly is to prevent
all motion of the blood from the heart and vena cava, whether it be
upwards towards the head or downwards towards the feet, or to either
side towards the arms, not a drop can pass; all motion of the blood,
beginning in the larger and tending towards the smaller veins, is
opposed and resisted by them; whilst the motion that proceeds from
the lesser end to end in the larger branches is favored, or, at all events,
a free and open passage is left for it.

WILLIAM HARVEY
de motu cordis.

It may be useful to think of veins as spaces as much as blood vessels,
despite their tubular shape and obvious transport function. In fact,
the venous system is commonly termed the capacitance system, re-
ferring to its reservoir function. The venous system is estimated to
contain as much as 60% of the total blood volume. Considering that
average venous pressure is still quite low (approximately 5–10 mm
Hg) it is clear that veins are quite distensible or compliant as compared with arteries; that is, much larger volume with only a fraction
of distending pressure. Veins do exhibit the property of flow resistance, to be sure, but in the absence of disease and at ordinary flow
rates it is negligible. For example, large changes in flow, such as those
accompanying exercise, occur with very little alteration in the capillary to right atrial pressure gradient. The reason for this is that the
capacity for venous flow is geared to maximal rather than minimal
flow rates. Therefore when the organism is at rest only a fraction of
the capacity is used. This is especially true of skeletal and cardiac
muscle veins. Under maximal flow, veins are fully distended and cy-
lindrical in cross section, but with less and less flow there is less and
less distending pressure and veins either assume an elliptical cross
section or they collapse to a variable degree. You can demonstrate
this with the superficial veins on the back of your hand using gravity
to alter distending pressure. Such passive alterations in flow conductance properties of veins render a different meaning to the concept of resistance than that intended. Quite clearly it would be wholly

inappropriate to infer alterations in venomotor tone to account for relatively high-calculated resistance values at low (resting) flow and low R at high flow (exercise).

VENOMOTOR TONE

The smooth muscle component in vein wall structure is very important to circulatory homeostasis because it permits regulation of the capacity of the venous system to suit particular physiologic circumstances, such as posture, exercise, and heart failure. By adjusting venomotor tone, potential discrepancies between venous return and cardiac output can be kept to a minimum. Venomotor tone, like arteriolar tone, is maintained by the complex interaction between vasoconstrictor and vasodilator influences. It would be both oversimplification and inaccurate to say that venomotor tone is qualitatively and quantitatively controlled the same way arteriolar tone is. In fact, while all agree the capacity for venoconstriction exists, some believe that the venous system is rather passive. Nonetheless, some similarities are recognizable such as sympathetically mediated basal constrictor tone. On the other hand, it is known that direct-acting vasoactive agents have quantitatively and even qualitatively different effects on veins as on arteries. In fact, an agent such as histamine, which is a powerful arteriolar dilator, seems to constrict veins. Furthermore, it seems that some agents, such as morphine, can relax venous while it seems to have little effect on arteriolar and constricts gallbladder smooth muscle. Obviously the physiology of smooth muscle is quite complex and our present knowledge of it incomplete.

EFFECT OF GRAVITY ON VENOUS CIRCULATION

The upright posture and the long distance from heart level to feet poses a serious problem for venous return. If the venous column was uninterrupted, the pressure in veins of the foot would be augmented by 100 mm Hg or more by the gravitational effect with attendant consequences for capillary fluid dynamics. Nature has dealt with this problem in a most ingenious way reducing its deleterious effect to a minimum.

The veins and lymphatic vessels of the extremities are equipped with valves (the functional purpose of which was so elegantly demonstrated by Harvey and so critical to his inference of the circulatory nature of blood flow). Venous valves by themselves serve only to give centripetal direction to blood flow and have only limited ability to obviate the long hydrostatic column. But the presence of valves in vessels surrounded by skeletal muscle or lying between the latter and a noncompliant integument is a different matter. Contracting muscles produce a compression of neighboring tissues which, because of valves, displaces blood in the veins and lymph in lymphatics toward the heart, reduces the magnitude of the vertical column and lowers venous pressure in dependent parts (Figures 8–4 and 10–1). This mechanism keeps the extent of vascular pooling and edema formation in dependent tissues to a minimum. Thus, skeletal muscle contraction represents an important source of energy for venous return, a source that becomes particularly valuable during exercise in the upright posture. Were venous and lymphatic valves not present, this energy source would be rendered ineffective because the compressive effect would result in undirected flow.

Veins above heart level in the erect posture have the opposite problem. The gravitational effect is to augment drainage toward the heart which, owing to lack of structural rigidity, leads to collapse of the veins. A collapsible tube cannot function as a siphon. Thus, collapse increases venous resistance and reduces the magnitude of gravitational effect on venous return from tissues above heart level. In addition, the tendency for pressure to be reduced in capillaries and veins in such tissues is minimized. A collapsed tube has totally different flow resistance properties than the same tube when it is partially or fully distended. Thus, capillary to right atrial pressure gradient remains fairly constant despite fluctuation in venous flow; a situation that renders uncertainty to calculated resistance.

Veins inside the skull and spinal canal are exposed to a totally different situation as regards distensibility or collapse. Assuming these spaces to be essentially fixed by the rigid boundaries and to be completely filled by essentially incompressible fluid contents, expansion or contraction of any component space (vascular, interstitial, or cellular) can occur only at the expense of equivalent change of opposite sign in another component unless pressure is to rise or fall markedly. In other words incompressible contents of a rigid container resist volume change. Thus in the head-up posture, the tendency for intracranial veins to collapse is prevented; this is translated to a siphoning effect on capillary flow so that the gravitational drop in

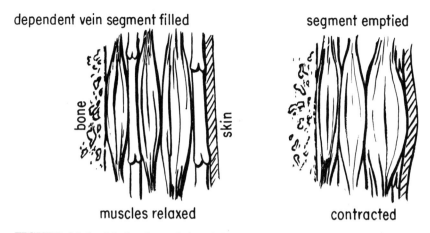

dependent vein segment filled   segment emptied

bone

skin

muscles relaxed   contracted

FIGURE 10–1 Mechanism of the skeletal muscle-venous valves pump for extremity venous return. This mechanism is particularly valuable during upright posture in man. On the left muscles are relaxed providing space for venous filling from below due to presence and orientation of valves. On muscular contraction, right, increased muscle volume impinges on soft tissue spaces obliterating veins and propelling blood cephalad due to valves.

arterial perfusion pressure is offset. In the head-down posture (or in the spinal canal below heart level in the upright posture), the incompressibility of contents confers equal gravitational effect on both arteries and veins such that the longitudinal pressure gradient remains fixed, a principle borrowed by the designers of so-called G suits to obviate extremity venous pooling during augmented gravitational forces of flight.

Thus far we have considered only two sources of energy for systemic venous return: the remaining potential (25–30 mm Hg) and kinetic energy of blood in capillaries provided by left ventricular contraction, and the milking action of skeletal muscle contraction on valved vessels. These energy sources have been termed *vis a tergo*, a push from behind. We will now consider sources that represent *vis a fronte*, a pull from in front.

THE RESPIRATORY PUMP FOR VENOUS RETURN

The pressure in the potential space in the thorax is normally subatmospheric during quiet breathing, waxing and waning with the phase of respiration. The reason is the chest cage, which is an elastic structure, and the inflated lung at the end of normal quiet expiration are held together (coupled) at a balance of opposing forces (i.e., the lung tending to collapse to its unstretched volume and the chest cage tending to spring out toward its resting position). In the supine position at this lung volume, intrapleural potential space pressure would be very nearly atmospheric. However, in the sitting or upright posture the effect of gravity on the fluid-like abdominal contents pulls the diaphragm downward and lowers intrapleural pressure slightly (i.e., makes it subatmospheric). Contraction of the diaphragm (i.e., inspiration) lowers the pressure even further, thus providing the pressure gradient for airflow from atmosphere into the alveoli. Subatmospheric intrathoracic pressure represents not only a force for air movement into the lung, it is also a force for blood flow from extrathoracic to intrathoracic veins, *vis a fronte*. This effect has been termed the respiratory pump for venous return since it waxes and wanes during the respiratory cycle, being more prominent during inspiration.

Finally, and only for the sake of completeness, another form of *vis a fronte*, ventricular diastolic suction, will be mentioned. In all probability this represents a negligible force for systemic venous return but it may promote pulmonary venous return. During ventricular contraction elastic elements of ventricular architecture are distorted such that energy is stored for subsequent recovery during diastolic restoration in the form of active early ventricular filling. The obvious analogy is a rubber syringe bulb used for aspiration. The relative structural rigidity of the left ventricle provides the potential for such an effect, but this is less likely as far as the right ventricle is concerned.

The heart pumps as a unit, but as far as the course of blood flow through it is concerned, the heart is two separate pumps connected in series with the pulmonary and systemic vascular beds interposed. Up to this point, we have talked about cardiac output and venous return as though there were only one of each when, in fact, because of the series connection, there are two. There are situations when it is downright misleading to talk about cardiac output or venous return without specifying which of the two of each one is discussing, for while they are inseparably linked, they also have independent determinants.

During steady-state conditions over extended periods the four variables are indeed equal or virtually so, but during transient periods there may be discrepancies that at times can be striking. Major discrepancies can exist for only brief transients, but small differences can persist for long periods. To the extent right and left ventricular outputs are unequal, so will venous returns be and a certain volume of blood will be transferred from one vascular bed to the other at a rate equal to the difference between the two flows (a precise treatment would have to take into account the fact that some bronchial blood flow returns directly to the left heart).

The combination of the skeletal muscle pump, regulatable venous capacitance, and the relatively large venous reservoir provide the possibility of a primary independent change in venous return initiating a change in cardiac output. In fact, this may be the only mechanism lower forms have at their disposal to alter cardiac output. There are situations where excessive venous pooling (either due to obstruction of major venous channels or to venodilatation) curtails venous return, hence cardiac output secondarily. This merely emphasizes Harvey's original discovery, that the "blood is impelled in a circle, and is in a state of ceaseless movement." Who can say where a circle begins or ends? Clearly, all factors that impinge on the system must be taken into account without dissociating what comes out of two pumps connected in series from what goes in.

LYMPHATIC SYSTEM

Despite its important and perhaps primary role in the body's defense against infection and other foreign substances, the lymphatic system is also considered a relevant part of the circulatory system because of its valuable transport function. It is appropriately included with the venous system because not only are lymphatics derived from veins, basically they serve the same general function: drainage of interstitial fluid. Lymphatics also provide an important avenue for transport of proteins and lipids into the circulation. The best way to illustrate the importance of lymphatic transport is to consider the consequence of experimental or disease-caused obstruction of lymphatic vessels. The effect is dramatic if the obstruction either is extensive or involves a major lymphatic duct. In the periphery (extremities), extensive lymphatic obstruction produces a very troublesome, occasionally massive and disfiguring intractable edema.

The lymphatic system begins as a network of blind-ended capillaries in the interstitial spaces of most tissues, exceptions including the brain and spinal cord. It ends in the thoracic and right lymphatic ducts that drain into large veins at the base of the neck. Along this path are scattered the lymph nodes through which lymph passes and is cleansed of harmful, especially infectious, material.

Total body lymph flow is not great by circulatory standards—approximately 2–4 liters/day in humans or 0.03% of the cardiac output. Obviously the flow in any particular lymphatic capillary is miniscule indeed. The reason for this should be readily apparent considering the pressure gradient from interstitial fluid to intrathoracic large veins.

As mentioned previously, lymphatic flow is aided by the same forces that promote venous return, the one striking quantitiative difference being the magnitude of intracapillary pressure. In lymphatic capillaries, there is no obligatory requirement for hydrostatic pressure to offset a high-plasma oncotic pressure. On the contrary, the formation of lymph requires that a net gradient exist from tissue fluid to lymphatic capillary. In terms of the Starling relationship, this raises questions as to the magnitude of tissue pressure and whether proteins enter lymphatic capillaries.

Both the composition of lymph and tissue pressure vary depending on the tissue and condition in which they are measured. However, the gross generalization can be made that tissue pressure, excluding gravitational effects, is of the order of a few mm Hg and thoracic duct lymph protein concentration something over half plasma concentration. Hepatic lymph protein concentration is quite high, almost as high as plasma, whereas that in lymph from the extremities is quite low, 1–2 g%. What this means is that the permeability of lymph capillaries is relatively great because water enters them despite a low pressure head and large protein and lipid molecules are able to enter as well. Thus, lymphatics provide a pathway for protein and lipid circulation and an alternative pathway for tissue interstitial fluid drainage which while quantitatively small is qualitatively of great importance. In circumstances where tissue pressure maybe elevated (e.g., dependency, venous disease, congestive heart failure, etc.), lymphatic circulation assumes even greater significance.

11
BLOOD VOLUME

... But indeed, supposing even the smallest quantity of blood to be passed through the heart and the lungs with each pulsation, a vastly greater amount would still be thrown into the arteries and whole body, than could by any possibility be supplied by the food and consumed; in short it could be furnished in no other way than by making a circuit and returning.

This truth, indeed, presents itself obviously before us when we consider what happens in the dissection of living animals; the great artery need not be divided, but a very small branch only, to have the whole of the blood in the body, as well of the veins as of the arteries, drained away in the course of no long time—some half hour or less. Butchers are well aware of the fact and can bear witness to it; for cutting the throat of an ox and so dividing the vessels of the neck, in less than a quarter of an hour they have all the vessels bloodless—the whole mass of blood has escaped.

WILLIAM HARVEY
de moto cordis.

The sea within us is comprised of the blood and interstitial fluid (i.e., extracellular fluid), for it is the constant exchange of all substances between these two compartments that determines the composition of the medium that bathes the cells of the body. The fact that cell water volume is more than twice that of interstitial water is impressive evidence of the efficiency of the exchange mechanism and gives some insight into how restricted the sea for each individual cell has become (Figure 11–1). Functioning in such a limited environment, it is small wonder that cell death follows so rapidly the termination of blood supply.

The blood volume in resting human beings is turned over approximately once each minute (5.0 liters at 5 liters/min). Since interstitial fluid is roughly six times plasma volume and the exchange of diffusible substances across the capillary membrane so free, the environment of cells is turned over about ten times per hour at rest. Turnover kinetics in the hummingbird must be many times faster; perhaps as much so as that during heavy exertion in humans when turnover increases several-fold. Turnover in the estivating lung fish and, to a lesser extent, in hibernating mammals, on the other hand, is markedly reduced.

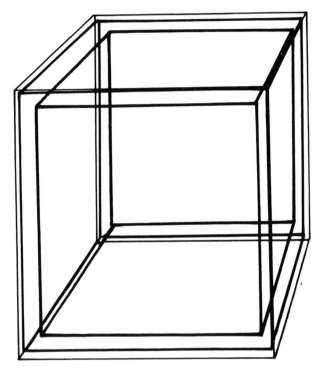

FIGURE 11–1 Distribution of body water among compartments. The blocks are drawn to approximate scale depicting relative water volumes of intracellular space (innermost block), interstitial fluid space (middle block less inner block) and plasma (outer minus middle block) showing how small the cellular environment volume is. This small volume in the face of high cellular metabolic activity is the basis for the high level of circulatory transport required to maintain homeostasis. The efficiency of circulatory transport and of diffusion may be inferred from the remarkably small plasma water volume (needed to suspend red blood cells) required to provide diffusion exchange.

DETERMINANTS OF BLOOD VOLUME

In general, a relationship exists between body size and blood volume among the species, but it is imperfect. It is hardly surprising that physically active species have a higher blood volume relative to body mass than do inactive ones. Even within a species blood volume is correlated with degree of physical activity. For example, augmentation of blood volume is an important aspect of the physiologic response to intensive conditioning (training) for competitive athletics. At the opposite extreme, marked reduction in blood volume (as much as 50%) accompanies hibernation (along with reductions in body temperature, metabolic rate, cardiac output, heart rate and blood pressure). Thus, not only is blood volume dynamic in the sense that it is in constant motion, it is dynamic in the sense that it fluctuates in quantity depending on demands placed on the circulatory apparatus to meet metabolic needs, or that the adequacy of blood volume plays a permissive role in the heart's ability to increase cardiac output in response to stress. Given the Frank-Starling mechanism, it should come as no surprise that one mechanism the body invokes to compensate for a failing heart is to increase blood volume above normal levels. Such volume augmentation, however, is not without secondary consequences, the ultimate effect of which may be self-defeating. This is discussed in greater detail in a subsequent chapter.

VASCULAR CAPACITY

The maximum capacity of the entire vascular system (all vascular smooth muscle completely relaxed) is substantially greater than the blood volume. Thus, what is called resting tone of vascular smooth muscle, a state resulting from the combined effects of inherent or myogenic tone, sympathetic α-adrenergic stimulation and the balance among all other direct vasodilatory and vasoconstriction influences, is responsible for keeping the potential discrepancy between vascular capacity and existing volume to a minimum. The arterial mechano-receptors and chemoreceptors (Chapter 12) serve the important, perhaps principal, role in this regard, but their effects are of limited duration so nature has developed other mechanisms that also have impressive survival value. Their ultimate purpose, as with mechano- and chemoreceptors, is to insure adequate perfusion of the brain, but they achieve this indirectly by effects that regulate body water, its distribution, and salinity.

REGULATION OF BODY WATER/BLOOD VOLUME

The amount of water in the body at any time is simply the steady-state balance between intake and loss and amounts to some 60–70% of body weight. There is usually only one source of intake, the gut, but many avenues of loss including gastrointestinal, renal, respiratory, and integumental. Assuming gain and loss to be equal, the steady-state balance point for water is that amount which in each species provides for physiologic osmolality of the cells. The regulatory mechanisms that achieve this are quite complex and they involve negative feedback systems (see Chapter 12) for control of thirst, salt intake, osmolality, blood volume, renal perfusion pressure, renal salt and water excretion, and gastrointestinal water loss. Because their effects tend to impinge primarily on the kidney, it is nigh impossible to discuss circulation physiology without touching on the renal role in blood pressure and, more especially, blood volume regulation.

Osmoreceptors and Antidiuretic Hormone (ADH)

In humans normal osmolality is represented by a solute concentration of 290–300 mOsm/kg. There are receptor cells in the anterior hypothalamus that somehow can detect a deviation (error signal) from this set point (threshold = 280 mOsm/kg) and set into motion effects that counteract the alteration. The receptors are called osmoreceptors (they are in or near the supraoptic and paraventricular nuclei) and they have nerve connections to neurohypophyseal cells of the posterior lobe of the pituitary wherein antidiuretic hormone (ADH) is produced and secreted. Increased osmolality (dehydration) causes osmoreceptors to stimulate ADH release and hydration (decreased osmolality) to inhibit it. The change in osmolality of plasma can be produced by any combination of imbalance between intake and/or loss of water and salt. Antidiuretic hormone is also called vasopressin or pitressin and it is an exceptionally, perhaps the most, powerful vasoconstrictor substance known, and yet, interestingly, its main effect is believed to be on the distal tubules of the nephron where by increasing permeability to water, water reabsorption is favored (i.e., antidiuresis) and a concentrated (hyperosmolar) urine excreted. In the absence of ADH, distal tubules being naturally impermeable to water, water reabsorption does not occur; therefore, a dilute urine is excreted. These effects, of course, would tend to correct the initial deviation in plasma osmolality because they represent imbalances in the relative amounts of water and salt retained (as well as excreted).

However, the osmoreceptor–ADH mechanism by itself cannot regulate total body water inasmuch as it can only sense and correct a concentration deviation. The ingestion or excretion of isosmolar fluid would change total body water and salt but would not change osmolality; thus the alteration would not be detected by the osmoreceptors. Nature has not left this loophole unplugged.

Low-Pressure (Volume) Mechanoreceptors

Evidence has been accumulated that suggests the presence of mechanoreceptors in heart chambers, especially the left atrium, which sense atrial volume (stretch) and have afferent connection via the vagus nerves to the ADH releasing mechanism. These have been called volume receptors or low-pressure baroreceptors and their negative feedback effect is to cause antidiuresis when atrial volume is low and diuresis when left atrial volume is excessive.

Renin–Angiotensin–Aldosterone System

Nature, not satisfied that she has designed sufficient redundancy of compensatory mechanisms to protect against distortions in the internal environment, came up with another ingenious system about which we have learned a great deal, but concerning which there is a lot more to know. It is called the renin–angiotensin–aldosterone mechanism and the history of the development of knowledge concerning it is fascinating.

Our present knowledge goes something like this: The so-called juxtamedullary apparatus of the afferent arterioles of cortical glomeruli in the kidneys contain and are capable of releasing into the circulation an enzyme called renin. From some set point pressure, decrease in afferent arteriolar pressure causes more renin formation and release whereas pressure elevation produces the opposite effects. Renin acts on a plasma protein called angiotensinogen or renin substrate to produce a decapeptide called angiotensin I. The latter is acted on by converting enzyme, primarily in the lung, which results in a powerful vasoconstrictor octopeptide, angiotensin II. Besides its direct vascular effect, angiotensin II has an additional well-documented effect and that is to stimulate release of aldosterone, the salt retaining corticosteroid, from the adrenal cortex. This hormone acts on the kidney to exchange hydrogen and potassium for sodium ion. Thus, the overall effect of the renin-angiotensin-aldosterone mechanism is to prevent blood pressure fall by maintaining blood volume through antidiuresis and salt (sodium) retention by the kidney and by direct vascular smooth muscle constrictor effect. The advantages of this system are that it does not depend on either the central or peripheral nervous system and its effect is long-lasting albeit slower on initiation. It is called into play by such stimuli as postural stress, dehydration, and possibly prolonged exercise. Recently it has been shown that angiotensin II when injected into the cerebral ventricles stimulates such things as drinking, ADH release, and sympathetically mediated hypertension. It is not known whether such effects occur physiologically because it appears that angiotensin crosses the socalled blood–brain barrier with difficulty, but there is now some evidence for a brain renin-angiotensin system.

Blood Volume and Cardiovascular Regulation

There are several disease states where both rapid and marked alterations in blood volume occur without a primary cardiac defect. These are interesting experiments of nature that provide important insights into what happens when blood volume regulation either fails or is overridden. There are acute inflammatory or toxic renal diseases wherein excretory function ceases (oliguria or anuria). Patients continue eating and drinking nevertheless and they usually present for medical attention when they notice soft tissue swelling or they have manifestations of high blood pressure (hypertension) or lung congestion. Similar manifestations occur in patients who inadvertently receive overzealous intravenous fluid replacement. At the opposite extreme are those clinical situations where blood volume is suddenly reduced, such as hemorrhage, severe diarrhea or vomiting, burns, dehydration, inadequate intravenous fluid replacement, or overzealous diuretic therapy. These commonly lead to hypotension (low blood pressure) or shock.

The conclusion to be drawn from such observations is that the blood pressure seems to rise and fall proprotional to body water balance, the two being linked through blood volume. The link between blood volume and blood pressure is cardiac output by way of venous return. What happens is that venous return increases as venous blood volume increases to the limit of venous vascular capacity without marked change in venous pressure. Beyond this, volume increments are accompanied by marked venous pressure increase as well, leading to congestion, at first peripheral but eventually pulmonary. Certain vascular beds such as the cerebral, coronary, and renal (Chapter 13), which account for half the cardiac output, resist overperfusion by a mechanism known as autoregulation. Thus, elevated cardiac output encounters a peripheral resistance that reflects a balance between vasoconstrictor and vasodilator influences, the latter mediated by baroreceptor reflexes (Chapter 11). Hypovolemia, on the other hand, leads to progressive disparity between venous blood volume and venous capacity. Veins collapse and venous return, hence cardiac output, falls. Autoregulation leads to certain vascular beds being vasodilated but central reflex mechanisms are stimulated by hypotension and hypoxemia, which tend to constrict others.

These phenomena are discussed as parts of the general clinical phenomena of shock and congestive heart failure (Chapters 15 and 16), but the important point is that blood volume is an integral part of the cardiovascular apparatus and its functional integrity is every bit as important as cardiac electric activity, Starling's law, peripheral resistance, etc. The important role of blood volume in cardiovascular regulation also can be gleaned from the number of mechanisms nature has evolved to assure its qualitative and quantitative integrity. These coupled with other mechanisms designed to keep vascular capacity appropriate to volume such that arterial pressure is maintained through both optimal venous return/cardiac output:total vascular conductance ratio provide the stability of the limited sea in which each and every cell in the body carries out its function.

12
CARDIOVASCULAR REFLEXES

The autonomic nervous system has been mentioned several times with regard to its role in the regulation of heart rate, stroke volume, and blood pressure. It is appropriate now to describe the components of this regulatory system and the mechanisms by which integrated physiologic adjustments occur in response to stresses such as posture and exercise and to various sensory stimuli.

Pacemaker potential produces cardiac automaticity (i.e., the heart beat) independent of extrinsic innervation and the length–tension (Frank–Starling), force–frequency (treppe) relationship and Anrep effect allow the heart to adjust total systolic energy output according to diastolic (loading) conditions without superimposed nerve-mediated inotropic effects. Thus, even in lower forms with so-called myogenic hearts, intrinsic cardiac adjustment to changing demands is possible but it is limited both in quantity and rapidity. This section deals with developments in higher organisms that provide for greater flexibility and speed in cardiovascular adjustment to increased demands.

PARASYMPATHETIC NERVOUS SYSTEM
AND CARDIOVASCULAR REGULATION

The development of parasympathetic (vagal) innervation of the heart represented a major evolutionary advance because it expanded the range of heart rate response to stress. Faster heart rates (achieved by reduced vagal depressor tone) coupled to increased venous return during temporary periods of increased cardiovascular demand provided a mechanism for increasing cardiac output without unduly large hearts to provide the cardiac component of increased oxygen transport required for greater muscle strength and endurance essential for mobility (successful forage, attack, defense, etc.).

If heart rate was to be determined by changing vagal tone, it is obvious that some regulating system was necessary to govern the latter. The control mechanism that developed, presumably over millions of years, is one that in modern engineering terms is referred to as a negative feedback control system. In complex higher organisms many such systems for controlling a large number and variety of physiologic variables have been identified, and undoubtedly there are many yet to be elucidated.

The basic components of a negative feedback control system include: (1) the controlled or regulated variable, (2) a mechanism (receptor) for sensing its quantitative deviation from a preset or predetermined optimal level (set point), (3) a mechanism for translating the error signal (deviation from optimal) into corrective response, (4) one or more effector mechanisms by whose actions the controlled variable will change (presumably for the better), and (5) communication links among these. The ingenious system that nature devised to regulate oxygen delivery by vagal heart rate control involves sensing both pressure and oxygen levels in blood perfusing the brain; not an unreasonable choice considering that the brain is the most important tissue in the body. Redundant mechanisms were added subsequently in complex higher forms for added flexibility and safety.

MECHANORECEPTORS AND CARDIOVASCULAR REGULATION

The more sensitive sentries of brain perfusion are the arterial mechanoreceptors located in the common carotid bifurcation (sinuses) bilaterally and around the outer curvature of the aortic arch. These receptors, innervated by cranial nerves IX and X bilaterally, respectively, are designed to detect changes in arterial blood pressure and their reflex effects are aimed at limiting, if not correcting, the change; hence, the synonyms of this mechanism: buffer, barostatic, modulator, baroreceptor, etc., reflex.

The receptors are sensory nerve endings in the walls of the blood vessels at these sites that generate action potentials as a function of both their static and dynamic deformation (hence mechanoreceptors), which depends on the degree and rate of change of distortion (stretch) of the vessel walls. Distention, in turn, varies both as a function of transmural distending pressure and vessel wall distensibility or compliance. Nominally, of all these factors, arterial blood pressure (BP) and its rate of rise will be the primary determinants of stretch receptor stimulation, but it is important to note that acute and chronic alterations in distensibility also may play an important role.

Mechanoreceptors are stimulated (i.e., generate afferent nerve impulses) beginning at a threshold pressure of 40–50 mm Hg increasing in a sigmoid relationship (this is called the transducer transfer function) plateauing at a blood pressure of about 200 mm Hg in experimental species in which it has been examined. The optimal value for BP (set point) obviously is the normal one in the resting animal not subject to stresses of any kind. This is approximately 80–90 mm Hg in humans. Deviations from this value represent errors that are sensed by the receptors leading to greater or lesser nerve impulse traffic in the buffer afferent nerves from some baseline level depending on whether pressure is higher or lower, respectively, than the set point value.

It should be obvious that the appropriate negative feedback response to afferent information arriving in the medullary integrative center in the brain must be to correct the error. This is how the term negative gets its significance. The appropriate compensatory response in every instance is qualitatively in the opposite direction (hence negative) to the original blood pressure error (change). Recall that BP is determined by only a limited number of variables: $SV \cdot HR \cdot \eta \cdot K/r^4$. Stimulation of mechanoreceptors by elevated blood pressure produces greater afferent nerve stimulus frequency which, in turn, stimulates central vagal nuclei resulting in heightened vagal cardiac efferent stimulus frequency. Cardiac vagal stimulation is inhibitory (i.e., depresses) because it slows SA node pacemaker frequency and depresses atrial contractile force. In mammals (possibly excepting hibernators) vagal innervation of the ventricles is rudimentary but in lower forms it is not. Thus, cardiac vagal stimulation reduces blood pressure by reducing heart rate primarily and secondarily by reducing stroke volume. It is possible that vagal stimualtion also depresses venous smooth muscle tone reciprocally. Such an effect would increase venous capacity, lower venous return, and contribute a peripheral component to decreasing stroke volume. A drop in carotid sinus and aortic arch pressure, such as occurs in assumption of the upright posture, produces opposite effects. However, it is important to note that while removing vagal depressor tone allows substantial cardioacceleration, it does not necessarily mean that cardiac contractile force is equally enhanced by diminished vagal tone. The latter effect in mammals is more dependent on reciprocal sympathetic activity and we will get to this momentarily.

The redundancy in baroreceptors represented by four separate (nerve) afferent inputs to the medullary integrating center provides insight into the biologic value attributed to this control system. The commonness and multiple etiology of human hypertension may be construed as evidence that nature evolved the system in mammals to protect against fall in blood pressure more so than rise. Thus, it is possible to infer that nature has treated hypotension as a more serious threat to survival of species than hypertension. In those species where high blood pressure is important for survival, she has provided heart, blood vessel, and control system with features that neutralize effects of hypertension that seem to be deleterious to animals with lower blood pressure.

DIVING REFLEX

The so-called diving reflex of aquatic animals provides insight into certain aspects of cardiovascular reflexes and is brought up here to illustrate that mechanisms other than baroreflexes impinge on the vagus. An air-breathing animal that has to dive underwater to obtain its meal is protected from the hypoxic effects of prolonged voluntary breath holding (30 min or more in whales and seals) by an amazing reflex, apparently hypothalmic, the effector output of which is characterized by oxygen-conserving, intense, generalized sympathetic vasoconstriction and vagally mediated pronounced bradycardia. Blood supply to the brain is assured because blood pressure is maintained while brain blood vessel bore is regulated primarily by CO_2 and O_2 tension in arterial blood rather than by sympathetic tone. Bradycardia (which can be abolished by atropine or vagotomy documenting its vagal mediation) reduces heart oxygen utilization to a minimum. Heart muscle blood flow is assured because coronary vasomotor tone is tied to myocardial O_2 demand. In effect, during a dive the animal becomes a heart-brain preparation as far as oxygen delivery is concerned, blood flow to all other tissues including skeletal muscle being severely compromised, forcing them to resort to temporary anaerobic glycolysis. It is some interest in this regard that exposure of certain fish (grunion, flying fish, mud skipper) to the air (air diving) also results in bradycardia. The diving reflex is rudimentary in man, but qualitatively the elements of the response are recognizable, including bradycardia, maintained blood pressure and peripheral vasoconstriction. It is clear the vagus can be stimulated to produce its depressor effects other than by stimulation of the mechanoreceptors. Vagal depressor responses are very easy to demonstrate in fishes, such as by stroking almost any part of their anatomy. So-called vasovagal attacks, characterized by bradycardia and hypotension and sometimes syncope (transient unconsciousness), are relatively common clinical occurrences that are mediated by a variety of sensor stimuli that are translated to a cortical input to the cardioinhibitory center.

The second system for regulating oxygen delivery to the brain is the oxygen-lack feedback system. The role of the oxygen-lack or chemoreceptors in cardiovascular regulation traditionally is considered to be minor, compared to their established role in respiratory regulation, but it is probably a lot more important than most people give it credit for. The reason is that its effects are brought out only by rather severe distortions; far beyond those that might be considered a part of everyday living. Thus, one way to think about it is that it represents a last line of defense; something that the body falls back on when all else has failed. If the mechanism saves a life in extremis, it would be a mistake to consider it unimportant in the total scheme of things. One occasionally hears of people coming back from the dead with or without apparently unsuccessful resuscitative efforts and while never documented to be the case, it is not impossible that the hypoxic mechanism provided the basis for survival.

CHEMORECEPTORS AND
CARDIOVASCULAR REGULATION

The so-called peripheral chemoreceptors are strategically located in a small glomus of nerve tissue in the bifurcation of both carotid arteries in mammals called the carotid bodies and in similar structures scattered about the inner arch of the aorta. They are innervated by the same nerves, IX and X, that innervated mechanoreceptors. (It is possible that there are central chemoreceptors in the brain itself). The high vascularity and blood flow of chemoreceptors previously alluded to means that their P_{O_2} is kept very high, essentially at arterial levels. Thus, the receptor cells are designed to detect even slight reduction in the P_{O_2} of their environment. How the chemical change is transduced into electrical signal output is not known.

Recall that in the earlier analysis of the factors that determined tissue P_{O_2} we made the reasonable assumption that a linear relationship existed between P_{O_2} and venous oxygen content (Cv_{O_2}). In the carotid and aortic bodies the extraordinarily high flow rate (2000 ml/ 100 g/min, estimated) means that there is essentially no arteriovenous oxygen difference. Thus, the venous value, hence tissue level, is on the flat (arterial) part of the sigmoid oxyhemoglobin dissociation curve (above 70 mm Hg) where small content changes are associated with large P_{O_2} changes. This makes the chemoreceptors very sensitive to factors which lower chemoreceptor blood flow absolutely or interfere with compensatory flow increase when arterial blood is hypoxemic for any reason.

The chemoreceptor afferent connections to cardiovascular integrative centers in the medulla are not as clearcut as to medullary respiratory centers. However, in circumstances where chemoreceptors are stimulated by low P_{O_2}, the primary effect seems to be slowing of heart rate and constriction of arterioles. While such effects are reminiscent of the diving reflex, it is not to say that the diving reflex is chemoreceptor mediated. The similarity of the decidedly paradoxical efferent output makes one wonder whether they don't share some mechanism in common. Vasoconstriction in the diving animal is sufficiently intense to maintain or even raise BP despite markedly reduced heart rate and cardiac output. We will come to hypothalamic control of cardiovascular effects shortly, but chemoreceptor or diving mediated vasoconstriction provide insight into how much more powerful the blood pressure compensatory mechanism can be when vessel bore changes also participate. This is especially true when the initiating stimulus is a fall in blood pressure. It is appropriate now to consider the sympathetic component of cardiovascular reflexes.

SYMPATHETIC NERVOUS SYSTEM
AND CARDIOVASCULAR REGULATION

The sympathetic nervous system is an ontogenetic as well as phylogenetic newcomer. It is apparently not fully developed in new born mammals while the vagus is. Most lower (marine) species do not have a sympathetic cardiac innervation although blood vessels may be. The development of the sympathetic system contributed significantly to greater flexibility and magnitude of motor responses because it provides a greater O_2 transport reserve and a means for its selective distribution.

The arrangement of vascular beds in parallel means, of course, that the distribution of cardiac output to the myriad of vessels will be determined by the relative resistances (or conductances) among them. Resistance is determined by the complex interaction of factors that regulate the tension of smooth muscle in the vessel wall of arterioles and percapillary sphincters, so-called vasomotor tone. It almost seems as though there is nothing in the body that doesn't have some effect on vascular smooth muscle tone under one circumstance or another. This applies to various ions, hormones, osmolarity, vasoactive peptides, enzymes, blood gases (O_2 and CO_2), and chemical mediators such as histamine, serotonin, prostaglandins, acetylcholine, angiotensin, vasopressin, epinephrine, and norepinephrine. With this array of potential controlling factors one would be a fool to look for a simplistic vasomotor control mechanism, but that mediated by the sympathetic nerves is the most important for temporary situations.

Lest the importance of parasympathetic control of certain blood vessels gets lost in the discussion of sympathetic control that follows, penile erection requisite for intercourse is a hemodynamic process that is mediated by parasympathetic nerves. Thus, survival of the species actually is more dependent on the more primitive parasympathetic division of autonomic nervous system.

Essentially all the blood vessels of the body are innervated by sympathetic nerves. The effect of sympathetic nerve stimulation is mediated by release of norepinephrine at the nerve terminus in effector tissues. The physiology of the sympathetic nerve terminal is quite complex. The mechanism by which a nerve impulse arriving at a nerve terminal (varicosity) releases norepinephrine is unknown, but as in the case of excitation–contraction coupling in muscle, calcium ion release seems to mediate the effect and is similar in many ways to neuromuscular transmission. It seems that there are a number of factors that can influence (inhibit) the norepinephrine release mechanism (so-called presynaptic receptors), and these include norepinephrine itself, angiotensin, acetylcholine, prostaglandins, and dopamine. Notice that these are naturally occurring substances that were included in the list of direct vasoactive substances. Thus, the complexity is that not only may they have an effect on smooth muscle tone directly, they have an indirect effect on sympathetic nerve-mediated tone by way of their influence on norepinephrine release.

ADRENERGIC RECEPTORS

Norephinephrine receptors in effector tissues are of two types, as judged by the fact that each can be selectively stimulated or blocked by certain drugs. The effects of cardiac sympathetic nerve stimulation were discussed previously, and they consist of increased frequency (chronotropy) and contractile force (inotropy). These effects of sympathetic nerves are designated those of β_1-adrenoreceptor stimulation, and they can be selectively stimulated or blocked by pharmacologic agents such as isoproterenol and propranolol, respectively.

Stimulation of sympathetic nerves innervating blood vessels causes vasoconstriction in most vascular beds except in the cerebral, coronary, and pulmonary, where effects are minimal. Such constriction is mediated by α-adrenoreceptor stimulation. However, certain vascular beds (skeletal muscle) as well as bronchial smooth muscle relax with sympathetic stimulation, a β_2-receptor effect. Furthermore, acetylcholine, the parasympathetic mediator, when injected into the pulmonary circulation causes pulmonary vascular smooth muscle to relax and bronchial smooth muscle to constrict! The mechanism for these different effects on the same tissue (i.e., smooth muscle) presumably has to do with whether excitatory or inhibitory effects are elicited and the types of receptors present. The vasoconstrictor effect of sympathetic nerve stimulation also can be selectively mimicked or blocked by pharmacologic agents such as methoxamine and phenoxybenzamine, respectively, agents which have no effect on β-receptors.

Cutting sympathetic nerves to blood vessels or pharmacologically blocking either ganglionic synaptic transmission or α-adrenoreceptors causes vasodilation. In the whole animal, α-blockade causes a fall in blood pressure by 10–30% if compensatory mechanisms are blocked. This means that sympathetic nerves are tonically active maintaining α-adrenergic basal smooth muscle constriction (vasomotor tone) in responsive vascular beds (skeletal muscle, splanchnic, renal, skin). This also provides the possibility for neurally mediated changes in vessel bore because tonic sympathetic activity can be withdrawn (vasodilation) or added to (further vasoconstriction). However, surgical or chemical sympathetic denervation does not result in complete smooth muscle relaxation. Substantial additional increase in tube bore (i.e., conductance) in these and other vascular beds can be demonstrated in response to a sufficient dose of many of the naturally occurring vasodilator factors previously mentioned such as vasoactive polypeptides, histamine, serotonin, prostaglandins, hypoxia, acidosis, and hyperosmolarity. These have a direct relaxing or paralyzing effect on vascular smooth muscle. In addition, there are several pharmacologic agents that share this type of depressor effect (e.g., sodium nitroprusside).

Thus, when vascular smooth muscle is completely paralyzed, the large pressure drop across the arterioles and precapillary sphincters is markedly reduced and blood pressure (at the same flow) falls to about a third of the normal value. One can infer from the foregoing that fully dilated blood vessels account for perhaps a third or more of total resistance, nonsympathetic intrinsic vascular tone about the same amount, and resting sympathetic tone the remainder. While the autonomic component of vascular control is complex because of α and β effects, it does have the singular advantage of rapidity of response, and on the constriction side it is potent. Thus, combined with the cardiac component previously discussed, potential fluctuations in blood pressure can be modulated in a matter of 10–15 sec. Persistent stresses challenging blood pressure homeostasis set into motion neurohormonal (pitressin) and hormonal (renin-angiotensin-aldosterone) responses that are slower in onset but longer in duration, relieving the autonomic mechanism of protracted requirement.

Having described the sympathetic system we can now briefly reconsider the barostatic reflex in terms of its total effects, components of which are shown in Figure 12–1. An increase in arterial pressure stimulates mechanoreceptors resulting in increased impulse traffic in afferent nerves IX and X. This information is received in the medullary cardioinhibitory (vagal) and vasomotor (sympathetic) centers, the first being excited while the second is reciprocally inhibited. The efferent outflow, therefore, is cardiac vagal stimulation which slows the heart, and decreases atrial contractility. Sympathetic outflow, on the other hand, is reduced; thus, α-adrenergic receptor stimulation in vascular smooth muscle, both arterial and venous, diminishes leading to vasodilation. Reduction in β-adrenergic cardiac stimulation results in less forceful ventricular contraction (i.e., reduced contractility). The net effect of all this is blood pressure reduction towards the

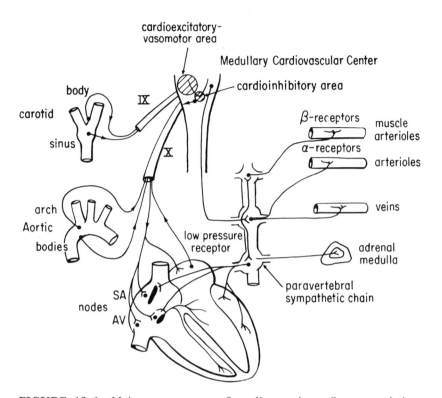

cardioexcitatory-
vasomotor area

Medullary Cardiovascular Center

cardioinhibitory area

body

carotid

sinus

IX

X

β-receptors

α-receptors

muscle
arterioles

arterioles

veins

arch

Aortic

bodies

low pressure
receptor

adrenal
medulla

SA

nodes

AV

paravertebral
sympathetic chain

FIGURE 12-1 Major components of cardiovascular reflex control (i.e., higher brain centers and local regulation excluded). Afferents from mechano- and chemoreceptors to medullary cardiovascular center via glossopharyngeal (IX) and vagus (X) nerves are shown. Efferent output is divided into vagal (parasympathetic) innervation of SA and AV nodes and atrial muscle and sympathetic innervation of heart, blood vessels and adrenal medulla.

set point level. A fall in blood pressure produces diametrically opposite effects.

The medullary level of cardiovascular integration is relatively simple compared to higher integrative centers in the hypothalamus or cortex. The diving reflex has already been alluded to. Everyone who has had an exciting or frightening emotional experience is aware of its effect on heart rate. Measurements show that contractility (cardiac output) and blood pressure increase in such circumstances as well; thus, a sympathetic discharge is clearly set into motion by emotions in the absence of a compromise either in cerebral oxygen supply or blood pressure.

This is only one example of how afferent information of a totally different character can be translated into cardiovascular effects emanating from the medullary centers. There are, of course, many others and they originate from and involve a variety of sensory input information and degrees of higher integration. Hypothalamic centers for temperature control and rage reaction have been localized, artificial stimulation of which can produce profound cardiovascular effects. Rushmer has performed elegant studies demonstrating a hypothalamic center, stimulation of which closely mimics the exercise response. Unlike the medullary level of integration, hypothalamic and other centers do not necessarily function by way of negative feedback. On the contrary, sometimes they set into motion effects that would get out of hand were it not for the modulating effect of the medullary negative feedback control of blood pressure. While the role of the medullary center in cardiovascular regulation has been appreciated for some time, we have only recently become aware of how complex and multifaceted the total central control mechanism is. Aside from the discovery of more and more reflexogenic centers in different parts of the brain and multiple interconnecting pathways, there is evidence which suggests the presence of central adrenergic, as well as central angiotensin mechanisms for blood pressure and blood volume regulation.

CARDIOVASCULAR RESPONSE TO EXERCISE

The conductance of regional vascular beds may change rather drastically under certain circumstances. These are detailed in Chapter 14, but they include effects such as hot environment on skin blood flow, hypoxia on cerebral or coronary blood flow, and digestion on splanchnic blood flow. Such conductance changes translate to cardiac output increases that keep the ratio CO/G, hence BP, constant. Dramatic as these may be in requiring an integrated cardiovascular response, they do not compare with adjustments that occur during heavy and prolonged muscular effort.

Skeletal muscle accounts for roughly half the body weight; thus, despite the fact that resting muscle blood flow is quite low, 3–5 ml/min/100 g, it still accounts for 15–20% of the resting cardiac output.

In an all out maximal muscular effort such as in athletic competition, cardiac output may exceed 30 liters/min for limited periods (the world record is about 40 liters/min), over half of this output supplying skeletal muscle (100 ml/min/100 g). In this circumstance, there is evidence that significant blood flow redistribution may occur such that inactive tissue (splanchnic, renal) blood flow is compromised to divert blood flow to skeletal and cardiac muscle. This diversion presumably depends on maximal generalized sympathetic vasoconstriction which in cerebral, cardiac, cutaneous and skeletal muscle is overridden by local vasodilatory determinants. Thus, the demands of severe muscular effort represent the greatest physiologic stress to which the cardiovascular system is exposed and while β-adrenoreceptor cardiac stimulation represents the cornerstone of the adjustments to these demands, α-adrenoreceptor vasoconstriction plays an important role too.

The overall or general control of the cardiovascular system is achieved by regulating cardiac output to maintain arterial blood pressure reasonably constant despite fluctuations of the myriad of individual conductances connected in parallel. The fact that blood pressure rises somewhat during most forms of exercise (and even strikingly so during isometric exercise) must mean that baroreflex resetting (decreased sensitivity) must be a part of the exercise response. Such a change could be explained on the basis of decreased distensibility of the mechanoreceptors in the carotid sinuses and aortic arch resulting from vascular smooth muscle contraction at these sites. Such vasoconstriction diminishes the degree of stretch of vascular wall and decreases the magnitude of distortion of the mechanoreceptors, a situation tantamount to a fall in blood pressure. This elicits a pressor response as well as tachycardia. Thus, the transducer transfer function is right shifted (i.e., equivalent to a resetting of the set point to a lower value). The higher blood pressure during exercise, therefore, is a response to mechanoreceptors that behave as though the blood pressure is lower than it actually is. A similar mechanism may be operating in the diving reflex due to the intense vasoconstrictive response; reflex tachycardia, however, is superceded by equally intense hypothalamically mediated vagal stimulation.

Patients with heart disease have a particular need for compensatory vasoconstriction when they exercise in the upright posture. When the capacity for cardiac output augmentation is limited because of heart failure, the increased conductance of the skeletal muscle vascular bed associated with exercise added to postural effects poses a serious competitive threat to cerebral blood flow. In this circumstance it is reasonable to expect that every available compensatory mechanism to preserve cerebral blood flow would be mustered and vasoconstriction would be among the more important in sustaining blood pressure. Chemoreceptor stimulation-mediated vasoconstriction may be the mechanism by which the mechanoreceptors are overridden to the extent that blood pressure is elevated during exercise even in patients with heart disease and failure. It is hardly surprising that in patients with severe heart failure (Chapter 16) blood pressure may fall during exercise.

A higher blood pressure associated with the marked increase in conductance of arteries supplying contracting skeletal muscle and in a more rapidly and vigorously contracting heart provides for greater oxygen transport to these tissues to satisfy their heightened energy consumption. But if all other tissue and organ vascular conductances were to remain unchanged (from that during rest) while BP increased, their individual flow rates also would increase. This is not what happens. As you might predict, cerebral blood flow is unchanged, skin blood flow increases except in severe exertion where it may decrease, and blood flow to most other tissues is variably decreased depending on the severity, duration, type, and stage of muscular effort. Vascular conductance in each tissue/organ is determined by the complex interaction of a number of general and local factors that impinge on vasomotor tone. Unselective sympathetic α and β adrenergic neurostimulation and circulating vasoactive substances such as catecholamines, angiotensin II, prostaglandins, polypeptides, vasopressin, etc., are included among the former, whereas local factors including P_{O_2}, P_{CO_2}, $[H^+]$, adrenosine, etc., are examples of the latter. The quantitative response of vascular smooth muscle to all such effectors cannot be assumed to be equal in all tissue (number and types of receptors), thus accounting for variability in individual tissue/organ conductance response.

The overriding importance of maintaining brain blood flow, whatever is happening elsewhere, is worthy of emphasis. Cerebral vessels respond to a number of vasodilators, both physiologic (P_{O_2}, P_{CO_2}, pH, histamine, bradykinin, etc.) and pharmacologic (alcohol, nitroglycerine, etc.), but they respond little, if at all, to sympathetic stimulation or circulating catecholamines. The ability of cerebral vessels to vasoconstrict, however, cannot be doubted since the phenomenon of so-called autoregulation is highly developed.

With so many factors having vasomotor potential, the logical question might well be asked whether an ordered controlling hierarchy exists among the various factors or mechanisms and, if so, what the order is. The complete truth undoubtedly is beyond our present limited knowledge, but certain insights are apparent. The diving reflex tells us that in species that depend on diving for food, sympathetic vasoconstriction can successfully override local factors in every organ save the brain and heart, at least temporarily. Clinical vasovagal syncope, a form of hypotension and low cardiac output often leading to transient unconsciousness (syncope) due to cerebral hypoperfusion, is mediated by a vagal discharge sufficiently strong that normal cardiac and peripheral vascular compensatory mechanisms are overridden. Anaphylaxis, a form of acute massive allergic reaction, seems to be mediated by the sudden release of large amounts of various vasodilator substances that override compensatory vasoconstriction but do not interfere with cardiac mechanisms primarily. Severe anger or anxiety can produce sporadic hypertension in man and other species demonstrating that the buffer reflexes can be overridden by inappropriate sympathetic stimulation from higher centers in the hypothalamus and cortex. Thus, it seems that while order usually prevails permitting an appropriate and integrated response such as in exercise, the system, presumably because of its complexity, occasionally can become discombobulated. To the extent that the negative feedback mechanisms are interrupted, the system either becomes aimless (uncontrolled), or worse, becomes a positive feedback system where an abnormality is perpetuated rather than counteracted.

EFFECTS OF CHRONIC CONDITIONING

It should be more evident now, especially in a trained athlete, why during exercise the heart is able to perform the prodigious amount of pressure–volume work previously mentioned. During training, the athlete's heart undergoes both dilatation and hypertrophy enabling it to accommodate larger end diastolic volumes without inordinate increase in filling pressure. Because of the large stroke volume, the heart is able to deliver normal resting cardiac output at a much slower

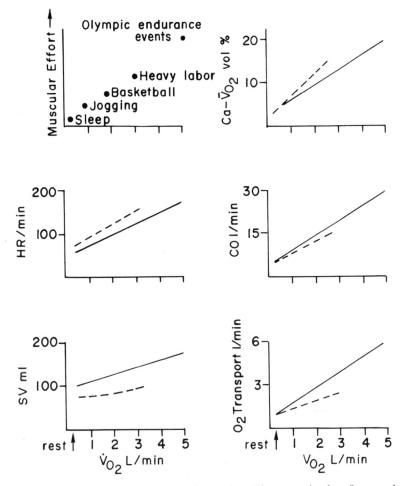

FIGURE 12-2 Hemodynamics of exercise. The magnitude of muscular effort is measured by the oxygen consumption as shown in the upper left. At rest (sleep) it is approximately 3 ml/min/kg body weight. During maximum steady-state exertion associated with competitive endurance events such as cross-country skiing, long-distance swimming and running as performed by world-class athletes (solid lines), it may reach 90 ml/min/kg or 6 liters/min. Incredible conditioning is required to achieve such levels of energy expenditure. The average person (dotted lines) would have difficulty reaching half as much and could do so for only brief periods. The differences in the two lines in each relationship represent the effect of prolonged vigorous conditioning: lower resting heart rate but higher maximum, larger stroke volume, tolerance of greater hypoxia (lower venous O_2 levels), higher cardiac output and O_2 transport.

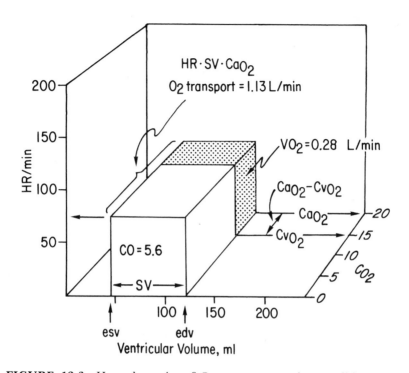

FIGURE 12-3 Hemodynamics of O_2 transport: resting conditions. Ventricular stroke volume (SV) is shown as difference between end-diastolic (EDV) and end-systolic (ESV) volumes. Cardiac output (CO) is product of SV and heart rate (HR). This area times arterial O_2 content (Ca_{O_2}) on the Z axis gives O_2 transport. Body oxygen consumption ($\dot{V}_{O_2}$) is 25% of this (shaded area) as determined by the arteriovenous O_2 difference.

heart rate. This is the physiologic resting bradycardia of athletic training so commonly observed. Training also increases the circulating blood volume, red blood cell mass and the capacity of the athlete to sustain higher heart rates during maximum effort. Thus, during exercise the athlete's heart is distended during diastole to a filling volume that provides optimal myofilament overlap for maximum number of interaction sites and maximal nerve mediated sympathetic β-adrenoreceptor stimulation, aided and abetted by high levels of circulating catecholamines secreted by the adrenal medulla, combine to produce maximal heart rate and positive inotropic stimulation. These

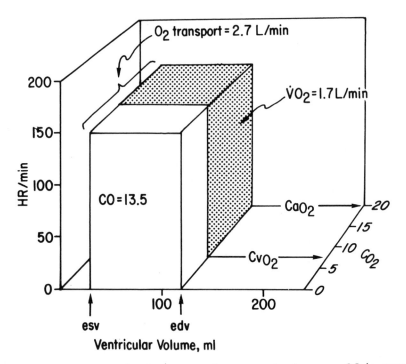

FIGURE 12–4 Exercise O_2 transport in an untrained person: CO increase achieved by heart rate increase. $\dot{V}_{O_2}$ increase by CO increase and greater arteriovenous O_2 difference (lower $C_{V_{O_2}}$).

plus the maximal length–tension effect make it possible for the heart to deliver as much as 30–40 liters of blood flow per minute at mean arterial blood pressure exceeding 100 mm Hg. Aside from all this, cardiac efficiency increases several-fold during exercise and the additional effects of greater red blood cell concentration and blood flow redistribution previously mentioned enhances even further the amount of oxygen that can be delivered to the vigorously contracting muscles. This explains how the twentyfold increases in oxygen consumption that have been measured in athletes are made possible by the hemodynamic component of the exercise response. The magnitude of this effect of conditioning in man is truly remarkable and estimates of its limits have had to be revised upwards several times in the past few decades because of superhuman performances of totally dedicated world-class athletes. These effects are depicted in

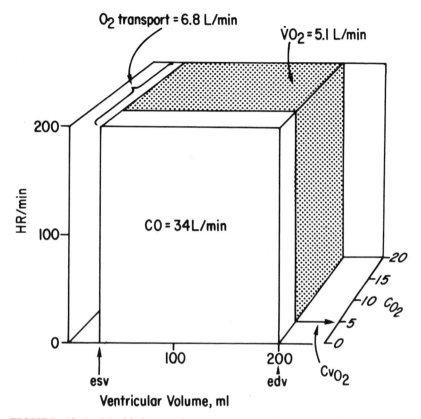

FIGURE 12–5 World-class endurance event athlete: markedly enhanced stroke volume, higher heart rate maximum and wider a-v difference providing huge $\dot{V}_{O_2}$.

Figures 12–2 to 12–5. Prodigious as such voluntary conditioning effects may be, they do not necessarily represent maximal development of cardiac energy output capability. Nature has conducted her own little experiments on this question and the results are astonishing. There are certain naturally occurring cardiac lesions that impose incredible burdens on the heart but are compatible with life. These conditions are present from birth and are superimposed on the usual demands of growth, development and voluntary activity (including athletics). There are many cases on record where these were all met without the patient being aware of a cardiac problem.

13

THE PULMONARY CIRCULATION

... transit is effected ... by the obscure porosities of the lungs and the minute inosculations of vessels. Whence it appears that, although one ventricle of the heart, the left to wit, would suffice for the distribution of the blood over the body, and its education from the vena cava, as indeed is done in those creatures that have no lungs, nature, nevertheless, when she ordained that the same blood should also percolate the lungs, saw herself obliged to add another ventricle, the right, the pulse of which should force the blood from the vena cava through the lungs into the cavity of the left ventricle. In this way, therefore, it may be said that the right ventricle is made for the sake of the lungs, and for the transmission of blood through them, not for their nutrition; seeing it were unreasonable to suppose that the lungs required any so much more copious a supply of nutriment, and that of so much purer and more spirituous a kind, as coming immediately from the ventricle of the heart, than either the brain with its peculiarly pure substance, or the eyes with their lustrous and truly admirable structure, or the flesh of the heart itself, which is more commodiously nourished by the coronary artery.

WILLIAM HARVEY *de motu cordis*

The emphasis up to this point on the systemic and no particular mention of the pulmonary circulation was not intended to imply that the so-called lesser circulation is less important. Indeed, of the capillary interfaces with the external environment in the skin, gut, kidney, and lung, that in the lung is undoubtedly the most important, for respiration, the uptake of oxygen and elimination of carbon dioxide by cells, represents the most fundamental of physiologic processes. The estivating lung fish can go without exogenous food and water or elaborating urine for fantastically long periods (up to 3 yr) but it does continue to breathe, albeit at a very slow rate, and circulation is maintained (heart rate of 1–3 beats/min).

The requirement for gas exchange brings essentially all the blood to within 1 μ of the external environment over a surface area that has been estimated to be 70 sq m approximately once each minute in man at rest. This exposure allows 250–300 ml of oxygen to be taken up and almost the same volume of CO_2 to be removed from the 5–6 litters of blood that perfuse the lung each minute. Obviously, the opposite processes (O_2 removal, CO_2 uptake) are going on at the same rate in blood perfusing the body tissues. The quantity of air that is breathed to allow the diffusion of gases to take place across the pulmonary alveolar–capillary membrane is variable depending primarily on the partial pressure of oxygen in the air which varies with altitude. As sea level, 3–4 liters of air are required to reach this membrane each minute. At this normal but relatively low level of alveolar ventilation, saturation of hemoglobin with oxygen is essentially complete but elimination of CO_2 is not, the partial pressure of CO_2 in blood falling from 46 mm Hg in mixed venous to 40 in arterial blood. However, this drop provides for elimination of 250–300 cc of CO_2 per minute. For 3–4 liters of gas to reach the gas exchange surface requires that 5–7 liters of air be breathed each minute, the amount depending on the pattern of breathing (frequency versus volume). Delivery of blood to this membrane in appropriate amounts to allow adequate gas exchange under all levels of activity and/or altitude exposure (consider mountaineers scaling peaks up to 26,000 ft without extra oxygen!) while satisfying certain critical hemodynamic requirements that we shall come to in a moment, presents remarkable design problems.

PULMONARY CAPILLARY DYNAMICS

A fundamental requirement of the pulmonary circulation is that the capillary hydrostatic pressure be kept well below that of colloid osmotic pressure, which is about 25 mm Hg. The reason for this requirement should be obvious. Recall that in body tissues generally it is important that net fluid movement between capillary and interstitial fluid be zero and that this is achieved by regulating capillary hydrostatic pressure to average 25 mm Hg to offset plasma osmotic pressure by the appropriate adjustment of pre- and postcapillary resistances, taking into account the flow. A similar situation in the lungs would be disastrous for the 1 μ alveolar–capillary membrane would not limit the liberal quantities of interstitial fluid thus made available from passing freely into the alveoli and destroying their gas transport function. This is because alveolar pressure, relative to circulatory pressures, for all practical purposes, is zero (i.e., atmospheric). Thus, as long as pulmonary capillary hydrostatic pressure is kept below plasma oncotic pressure, the force for fluid reabsorption will exceed that for filtration and the alveoli will remain dry. To maintain pulmonary capillary hydrostatic pressure at low levels while satisfying the filling pressure requirements of the left ventricle and at the same time accommodating flow increases up to four- to fivefold during exercise presents real problems.

To begin with, energy requirement for filling the left ventricle comes largely from the pumping action of the right ventricle. The relaxed or diastolic distensibility characteristic of the left ventricle is such that at physiologic heart rate in man at rest an average left atrial pressure of about 5 mm Hg is required to deliver a physiologic stroke volume to the left ventricle during diastole. Thus, even if there were no pressure gradient associated with pulmonary venous flow (a physiologic impossibility) the lowest pulmonary capillary pressure could be is 5 mm Hg. In general, left atrial pressure rises as cardiac output increases because of the Frank–Starling mechanism despite the operation of factors that are designed to keep left ventricular filling pressure down, such as increased heart rate, greater ventricular emptying and enhanced myocardial contratility. In fact, at maximum cardiac output levels associated with severe exercise, left atrial pressure may approach and even reach 25 mm Hg, especially in certain parts of the lung, and this may be the factor which limits the exercise tolerance of certain athletes or individuals whereas in others the limiting factor is respiratory. In any event, the pressure requirement for filling the left ventricle represents the floor below which pulmonary capillary pressure cannot be, whereas the ceiling is represented by the colloid osmotic pressure of plasma above which filtration exceeds reabsorption and alveolar spaces become filled with fluid, a condition known as pulmonary edema. The fact that there is both a floor and a ceiling and that the floor rises toward the ceiling as cardiac output increases represents some of the problems peculiar to the pulmonary circulation. There are others.

As we have already seen, man's assumption of the erect posture has resulted in problems with regard to capillary dynamics in and venous return from dependent parts and to arterial circulation to tissues above heart level. It has created problems for pulmonary circulation as well.

PRESSURES IN THE PULMONARY CIRCULATION AND EFFECT OF GRAVITY

The main pulmonary artery branches are located and arborize in such a way that about half the lung is superior and half inferior to them when man sits or stands. The gravitational effect from this midpoint to top and bottom is opposite in sign, being negative for blood flowing upward and positive for blood flowing downward. The difference in gravitational hydrostatic pressure from top to bottom amounts to some 20 mm Hg. This means that whatever the pressure is at the midpoint, it is about 10 mm Hg less than this at the apex and, conversely, 10 mm Hg more at the base of the lung (Figure 13–1). The pressure decrement or increment has the obvious effect

FIGURE 13–1 Pulmonary circulatory pressures at various sites and effect of gravity. Note higher pressures in vessels at lung base and low distending pressures in apical vessels. Apical veins and capillaries potentially or may actually collapse but negative intrapleural pressure would help keep them open. In the basal capillaries pressure approaches plasma oncotic level unless arteriolar constriction imposes a pressure gradient (dotted lines) lowering capillary pressure.

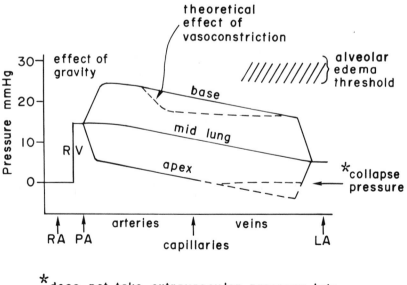

*does not take extravascular pressure into account

of making the bore of vessels respectively less than or greater than those at the midpoint not under positive or negative gravitational influence, relatively speaking. Thus, whatever the overall flow resistance of the pulmonary circulation in the erect posture, the gravitational effect would make it lower in the lower half of the lung than in the upper unless there is a mechanism to counteract this effect. We will develop this further subsequently, but first we need to examine the general pressure–flow relationships in the pulmonary circulation.

The requirement of a low pulmonary capillary hydrostatic pressure could be achieved by having a very low arterial pressure and no intervening resistance or a higher arterial pressure with an appropriately graded precapillary resistance which would reduce the pressure before it reached the capillaries as in the case of the systemic circulation. The advantages of the former are two-fold: (1) Because it would be a passive system, changes in flow would require no regulating system; and (2) it would require the least pressure-volume work on the part of the right ventricle to perfuse the lung since there would be no added resistance to overcome. The second option has no advantage as far as pulmonary circulation is concerned under normal circumstances except one: It represents a neat mechanism for shutting down the pulmonary circulation in the fetus where such circulation is not needed. In fact, the resistance to blood flow of the fetal lung is higher than that of the body and this causes most of the oxygenated umbilical vein blood to bypass the lung by shunting through various defects (i.e., atrial and ventricular and the patent ductus arteriosus) into the left heart. So it seems that despite the fact the design is not favorable for life post partum, it is important to have a high precapillary pulmonary vascular resistance before birth.

Studies in the newborn sheep have demonstrated that with the onset of breathing, the initially high fetal pulmonary artery pressure (60 mm Hg) falls rather precipitously despite the fact that pulmonary blood flow is increasing rapidly during this same period. This means that the high resistance in the precapillary pulmonary vessels evaporates within minutes! Studies, even in human newborns, have demonstrated rapid decrease in pulmonary artery pressure, but it is more gradual, the adult level being reached in days instead of hours. There is morphologic evidence in terms of the marked hypertrophy of the media (smooth muscle layer) of small pulmonary arteries that exists

in utero and disappears after birth that corroborates these hemodynamic events. Thus, nature takes advantage of both options, a high-
resistance system for in utero and low resistance one for the rest of
life. It might be appropriate to mention here that nature does make
mistakes, for once in a while the high resistance fails to recede and
such a person is stuck with a high-pressure pulmonary arterial system
for life. At the same time, there are congenital cardiac lesions in
which persistence of the fetal high-resistance pulmonary circulation
is mandatory for life.

Normal pulmonary artery mean pressure in supine resting man is
about 15 mm Hg and left atrial pressure 5 mm Hg. This means the
resting cardiac output is pumped through the lungs with a pressure
gradient of only 10 mm Hg, a remarkable contrast with the systemic
circulation; in terms of resistance, $R = \Delta P/\dot{Q} = 10/6 = 1.67$ mm Hg/
liters/min for the lung versus $90/6 = 15$ mm Hg/liters/min for the
body. This 10 mm Hg pressure gradient is distributed fairly evenly
across the large and small arteries, capillaries, and small and large
veins. This means that hydrostatic pressure at the capillary midpoint
is between 5 and 10 mm Hg, a value well suited for maintaining dry
alveoli.

Recall, however, that in upright man there is a 10-mm negative
pressure head to overcome for blood to reach the apices of the lungs.
Assuming that the left atrium is at the midchest level (which it is not)
and assuming no other factors operating, this means that the arterial
pressure at the top of the lung would be 5 mm Hg and capillary
pressure zero. Transmural venous pressures in the apices could even
be negative resulting in their intermittent collapse. Obviously, the
flow at this level would be markedly reduced. At the opposite extreme
the vessels in the most dependent part of the lung are subjected to
arterial pressures up to 20–25 mm Hg and would carry far more than
the average flow. This is shown in a schematic model (Figure 13–2)
which illustrates some of the theoretical complexities of the situation.

The situation depicted has several unusual features:

1. It shows a horizontal arteriovenous pressure gradient of 10 mm
Hg at each level despite the variation in the size of the arteriovenous
pathway. Pulmonary vessels are thin-walled and rather distensible;
furthermore, they are surrounded by very low pressure, perhaps
even negative. Thus, vessels under high-intraluminal pressures will
be distended and those under low pressure will be narrow (this is

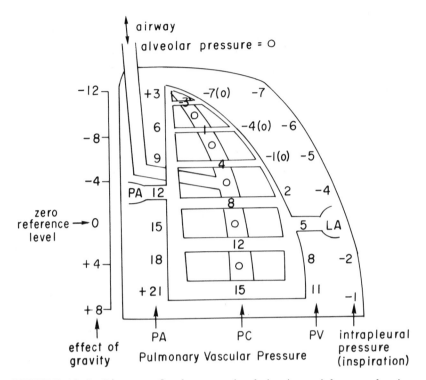

FIGURE 13–2 Diagram of pulmonary circulation in upright man showing effect of gravity on vascular pressures and alveolar and intrapleural pressures on distending (transmural pressures). Explained in text.

shown by the width of the tubes). It should be obvious that the larger tubes will carry vastly more flow ($\dot{Q} = K r^4$), pressure gradients being equal.

2. The capillaries in the upper one-third of the lung would be collapsed part of the time at the venous end of the alveolus because they are under negative transmural pressure (i.e., atmospheric pressure in alveolus, subatmospheric pressure in capillary). However, as long as pulmonary arterial pressure is high enough to overcome the negative gravitational pressure and get the blood up to the capillaries in the top third of the lung it will flow. However, it will flow intermittently, for such a system functions as a flutter valve in which considerable energy is "wasted" in accelerating and decelerating blood since it starts and stops cyclically. Another factor that may be of some importance with regard to the negative hydrostatic pressure head in

the upper veins is negative intrapleural pressures. Note that by adding to the transmural distending pressure across the walls of both
arteries and veins, it distends them without contributing to the arteriovenous flow gradient. In the upper part of the lung, it helps keep
veins open. It should be pointed out that intrapleural pressure is not
uniform throughout the potential pleural space; because the lung
tends to hang in the thorax due to gravity, intrapleural pressure is
more negative at the apex compared to the base.

3. The worst feature of this situation is the high-capillary pressures in the lowest third of the lung. The ones shown are still below
plasma oncotic pressure but they are too close for comfort in that
they provide no reserve margin from the development of lung
edema. One counteracting factor is the vertical location of the left
atrium and the effect of gravity on left atrial pressure. In the upright
human, the left atrium is actually a posterior structure that lies below
the level of the backward-arching main pulmonary artery, its horizontal midpoint being 3–4 cm lower. Thus, true intravascular pulmonary pressures may be lower by this amount. Upright posture also
has an effect on cardiac output and blood volume distribution. The
CO is lower in the sitting than supine and lower in the quiet standing
than sitting position. The reason for this is that blood, as much as
500 ml of it, shifts from upper, including thorax, to dependent parts
(i.e., it pools). Intracardiac volumes and diastolic pressures, accordingly, are reduced resulting in a lower cardiac output due to the
Starling (length–tension) effect. Thus, left atrial pressure in the upright posture is a few to possibly several millimeters of mercury less
than in the supine position.

It is unthinkable that nature would overlook the problem of high
capillary pressures at the base of the lung. One solution is rather
obvious: place graded precapillary resistances in the lower half of the
lung to lower the pressure. The lower limit to which capillary pressure could be reduced by this means is the venous pressure at each
level, or 4 mm Hg less than what is shown at each level. While such
resistances would reduce flow at the same overall pressure gradient
compared with the supine situation, it would not matter, for the erect
posture has the effect of reducing cardiac output as a consequence
of systemic venous pooling anyway.

To summarize, the adult human pulmonary circulation has a remarkably low resistance owing to the rapid regression of the con-

stricted and/or hypertrophied medial smooth muscle present in the fetus. Assumption of the erect posture which results in qualitatively and quantitatively different gravitational forces on the blood depending on whether it is in vessels above or below the entrance–exit level, results in uneven flow distribution (top < bottom) that may be partially compensated by retention of precapillary resistance in the lower half of the lung. Such resistance has the more important effect of reducing high capillary pressures in the dependent portions.

PULMONARY BLOOD FLOW CAPACITY

How then does the pulmonary circulation manage the flow increases associated with exercise? Some insight can be gained by certain observations that illustrate dramatically how low resistance in the pulmonary vessels is and can be:

1. Sudden occlusion of the left or right main branch of the pulmonary artery with a balloon-tipped catheter has no effect on cardiac output (it is all diverted to the unoccluded lung) and raises pulmonary artery pressure only a few millimeters of mercury (the maneuver has no noticeable effect on a conscious subject). Thus, resistance in the unoccluded lung essentially halves and it demonstrates the reserve capacity of the pulmonary circulation. Under resting conditions only a fraction of the lung vascular bed need be in use and explains why patients can tolerate pneumonectomy (removal of one lung).

2. In certain congenital cardiac lesions, wherein a large volume of blood recirculates through the lung without perfusing the body, pulmonary blood flow may be 25–30 l/min at rest! Such lesions may not represent a reasonable model of an Olympian going flat out in competition to achieve a similarly high level of cardiac output (the left ventricle does not participate in the high flow), but such patients are a lot easier to study. At any rate, such flows have been measured, associated with a mean pulmonary artery pressure of as low as 25 mm Hg! Pulmonary overcirculation in such patients obviously has adapted gradually since birth, but perhaps so have the athlete's during the long period of rigorous training. These exceptional situations admirably demonstrate that flow increases can be accommodated without excessive pulmonary vascular pressures. It was indicated previously in what way exercise imposes an additional requirement on the pulmonary circulation which make these observations only par-

tially relevant and make maintenance of a low capillary pressure more difficult. Be that as it may, pulmonary blood flow increases associated with ordinary exercise occur with only modest increments in pulmonary arterial pressure. Presumably this is owing to recruitment of closed as well as expansion of existing vessels in the high-capacity bed.

PULMONARY VASOMOTION

Until quite recently, the pulmonary vascular bed was thought to be completely passive (i.e., that the vascular smooth muscle while present served no function or role). There is convincing evidence now that the pulmonary vessels constrict under certain conditions. Most important among these from the physiologic point of view is the pulmonary arterial constriction associated with inhalation of air or gas mixtures containing low oxygen partial pressure and with chronically elevated pulmonary capillary–venous pressure. The vasomotor responses of gill arches in teleosts and elasmobranchs provide insight into pulmonary vascular responses in higher organisms. For example, it has been shown that vagal stimulation constricts and catecholamines dilate branchial vessels, effects which can be blocked by atropine and propranolol, respectively. Propranolol, the β-adrenoreceptor blocker, itself causes branchial constriction, consistent with the interpretation that tonic β-receptor stimulation branchial dilation is present. The catecholamine effect, therefore, is a beta, not alpha effect. The significance of this is that qualitatively similar effects have been found in mammalian pulmonary circulation. For example, while an α-adrenergic pulmonary vasoconstrictor effect has been demonstrated with norepinephrine, it is weak; whereas the vasodilator effect of isoproterenol (β-receptor stimulation) or acetylcholine (the vagal mediator) are relatively potent, especially when pulmonary artery pressure is elevated. Also, propranolol β-blockade causes bronchoconstriction and possibly pulmonary vascular constriction. Thus, the phylogenetic thread does seem traceable even though the mammalian pulmonary vessels have evolved to a relatively inactive state from the standpoint of vasomotor reactivity.

Acute or chronic hypoxic pulmonary vasoconstriction has been demonstrated to occur in a number of species including man; however, the magnitude of the response varies considerably within and among species. The reasons for these differences remain unknown. The survival value of such a response is elusive, but one possible explanation is that it represents an attempt on the part of the body to redistribute the pulmonary blood flow in such a way that a greater fraction perfuses upper segments of the lungs. This would have the beneficial effect of improving what is referred to as the ventilation-perfusion ($\dot{V}_A/\dot{Q}$) relationship. Recall that in the upright posture the upper third of the lungs is relatively underperfused while the lower third is overperfused. Another way of saying the same thing is that relatively the upper one-third is overventilated and the bottom one-third underventilated. These situations waste both ventilation (in the upper one-third) and perfusion (in the lower one-third). Anything that makes for a better balance between the two physiologic parameters will make for more efficient gas exchange and this would be especially desirable under hypoxic conditions. Pulmonary vasoconstriction, especially if it were to occur predominantly in the lower one-half of the lung, would accomplish this by raising arterial pressure. The higher arterial pressure and the greater arterial (precapillary) resistance in the lower parts represent a standoff, the first tending to increase flow, the latter tending to decrease it. Thus, flow in the dependent portions of the lung might be unchanged. However, in the upper segments of the lung, the higher pressure provides an adequate perfusion gradient to overcome the negative gravitational effect on the arterial side. The greater transmural pressures in the capillaries or venules in turn would tend to keep them open and allow the siphon effect of negative venous pressure to operate more effectively. It is likely that these effects would more than compensate for the effect of vasoconstriction and result in greater flow reaching the upper, well-ventilated alveolar–capillary membrane.

There are many disease conditions that result in elevation of pressures in the left atrium, pulmonary veins, and capillaries. Most of these are due to left ventricular failure, but mitral valve stenosis (narrowing) is the most dramatic prototype. Such pressure elevation upsets what at best is a marginal situation in the base of the lungs, a capillary–venous pressure of approximately 10 mm Hg. Additional elevation of this pressure makes the basal portion of the lung vulnerable to pulmonary edema. Again, peripheral pooling in the upright posture ameliorates this tendency. Pulmonary arterial vasoconstriction, especially in basal vessels, also would improve this situation by reducing flow to the bases and shifting flow to the upper lobes. There is radiographic support for a mechanism of this type commonly referred to as redistribution of flow to the apices associated with left heart disease. Thus pulmonary vasomotion can be said to have survival value. Unfortunately sometimes it gets out of hand and itself becomes a primary problem. For example, in chronic hypoxemia in man and in certain animal species and in chronic elevation of left heart pressures associated with mitral stenosis or left ventricular failure, the pulmonary vasoconstrictive response may become so exaggerated in certain cases that resulting pulmonary arterial hypertension becomes pathologic rather than physiologic, leading as it does to chronic right heart failure.

The benefits that accrue from such pulmonary vasoconstriction responses are not without cost to the organism. It is on the right ventricle that the increased workload of generating a higher pressure falls. It is appropriate, therefore, to consider some of the special features of the right ventricle which has the functions of providing the energy to get systemic venous return through the lung and to load the left ventricle.

RIGHT VENTRICULAR DYNAMICS

The hemodynamic features of the pulmonary circulation are important to the right ventricle, for they determine the pressure that it must generate during systole which, in turn, determines the wall tension necessary. The right ventricle is said to be better suited for volume pumping than for pressure pumping. What is meant by this is that the right ventricle is well-equipped to eject its volume efficiently but is poorly designed to generate pressure, whereas with the left ventricle it is just the opposite. The left ventricular myocardium has the shape of a rounded cone, the wall of which is thickest at the base where it measures 10–12 mm and gradually thins out toward the apex where it is only 2–3 mm. The right ventricle appears to be attached to the anteroright lateral surface of the base of this cone forming a cavity of two concentric arcs, the smaller internal one being that of the outside of the cone (septum) and the larger outside one being that of the right ventricular free wall (Figure 13–3). A given amount of shortening of the contractile element or sarcomere will have greater effect on volume change within the chamber when the

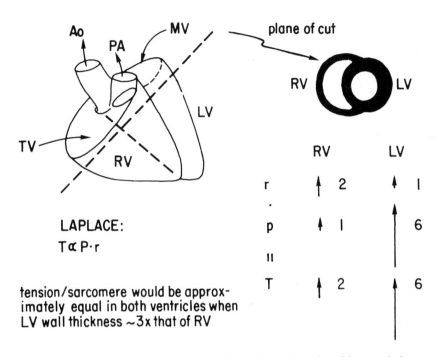

FIGURE 13-3 Relationship between hemodynamic and architectural characteristics of left and right ventricles. Ventricular wall thickness reflects wall tension at that point as determined by Laplace relation. Grossly (ignoring complex architecture and wall thickness itself) the ratio is 3:1, LV:RV.

radius of curvature of the arc is large than when it is small. On the other hand, the larger the radius of curvature, the more tension is required to effect the same intraventricular pressure. The latter is a statement of the law of Laplace: Tension α pressure × radius. Applied to the left ventricle it illustrates the mechanical principle behind the anatomic observation that the left ventricular wall is very thin at the apex where the average radius of curvature is small and thickest at the base where the average radius is large despite the fact that the intraventricular pressure during systole is the same throughout. Obviously where the radius is large a great deal more tension is required for a particular pressure and this requires a lot more fibers if each unit creates the same tension regardless of the radius. To get back to the right ventricle, its larger radius of curvature places it at a disadvantage in generating high pressure, but since ordinarily the low resistance pulmonary circulation spares it from meeting this requirement, it becomes clear why the right ventricular wall is thin (2–4 mm) throughout and geared for ejecting its volume efficiently.

Therefore, it can be argued that the thickness of ventricular wall varies directly with the tension work it is required to perform at that location. A corollary of such a conclusion is that each cardiac sarcomere develops essentially the same tension during contraction as every other sarcomere regardless of location in atrium or ventricle, in the left or right side and in apex or base. Wall thickness accurately reflects the magnitude of this tension work. This may explain why the heart has a way of knowing how to adapt to requirements placed upon it. When the systolic tension-generating requirement is high, such as is normally the case for the base of the left ventricle or associated with pathologic processes that result in elevation of ventricular systolic pressure, the heart responds by laying down or elaborating more fibrils (i.e., it hypertrophies). This situation is comparable to the massive development of skeletal muscle mass by athletes who train for a sport that involves primarily isometric contraction (e.g., weightlifting). On the other hand, when the requirement is for greater volume change of the ventricular cavity between end diastole and end systole, i.e., greater fiber shortening, the chamber dilates but hypertrophies relatively less. This is comparable to the lesser degree of muscular development in athletes who engage in sports that require endurance or repetitive isotonic contractions rather than strength, e.g., long-distance running, or the heart responds to high levels of isometric work by increasing muscle mass (hypertrophy) and to increased isotonic work by greater resting length (dilatation). These two responses are at cross purposes. In certain cardiovascular disease one or both ventricles may be confronted with both requirements simultaneously. As could be predicted, the heart tolerates such situations poorly and rapidly fails. The right ventricle is particularly prone to fail in the face of a pressure load, particularly if that load has not been present from birth.

14

SPECIAL FEATURES OF CERTAIN VASCULAR BEDS AND HYPOXEMIA

CEREBRAL CIRCULATION

The brain is unquestionably the most important organ in the body and it is wholly dependent on aerobic metabolism for its function, the higher cortical neurones being especially sensitive to the slightest degree of hypoxia, unconsciousness reflecting its presence. It is hardly surprising, therefore, that elaborate and redundant external and intrinsic mechanisms evolved to assure constant oxygen supply to the brain. In man cerebral blood flow averages about 50 ml/min/ 100 g and constitutes about 15% of the cardiac output. This level of cerebral perfusion is such that venous blood oxygen content is slightly lower than of the body average. Since brain oxygen consumption is remarkably constant, varying hardly at all between sleep on the one hand and mightly thought or worry on the other, a constant cerebral blood flow will satisfy most conditions of constant O_2 transport. However, a fall in arterial blood O_2 content, Ca_{O_2}, such as in hypoxemia or anemia, can be compensated for only by an increase in flow. The fact that blood pressure is regulated means that such flow increases depend on cerebral vasodilatation. (Recall the two equations: O_2 transport $= Ca_{O_2} \times$ blood flow and tissue $P_{O_2} \propto Ca_{O_2} - \dot{V}_{O_2}/\dot{Q}$).

The mechanisms that are strategically located to assure cerebral blood flow include: the carotid and aortic mechanoreceptors and chemoreceptors that elicit a sympathetic discharge whenever brain blood flow is threatened (i.e., by a fall in blood pressure), possible central chemoreceptors in the brain itself, and the ADH and renin–angiotensin mechanisms that insure adequate vascular volume at all times.

The special features of cerebral circulation include: (1) the location of the brain inside the rigid skull, which minimizes gravitational forces from affecting cerebral blood flow; (2) vascular smooth muscle largely unresponsive to α-adrenergic neuro- or chemostimulation but highly responsive to hypoxemia and hypercapnia; and (3) blood flow autoregulation. The consequence of these mechanisms is the same monotonous theme, they guard against compromise of brain oxygen supply.

Consider the threat to cerebral oxygenation of mountain climbing at elevations above 25,000 ft without supplemental O_2 (this actually has been done in the Himalayas). At this high altitude, the P_{O_2} of air is approximately 60 mm Hg, a marginal value for survival because it is reduced even further (to about 45) by the effect of water vapor (47 mm Hg) and P_{CO_2} (approximately 30) additions in the lungs encroaching on P_{O_2}. Climbs at this level are impossible without maximal acclimatization which produces cardiopulmonary adjustments, polycythemia (to increase Ca_{O_2}) and development of brain and tissue tolerance to effects of chronic hypoxia and hypocapnia. Chemoreceptor-mediated hyperventilation (to maximize P_{O_2} but at the expense of reduced P_{CO_2}) at high altitude creates confusing biochemical signals to cerebral vessels, hypoxia to dilate, and hypocapnia and alkalosis to constrict. That dilatation occurs is proof positive which is the more compelling stimulus. When the first conquerors of Everest, Hillary, and Tenzing, (and others have done since) took off their O_2 masks on the top of Mt. Everest (ambient P_{O_2} = 50), their cerebral and coronary blood flows must have been prodigious. Equally dramatic are patients with chronic severe pulmonary disease who somehow manage to function with arterial blood P_{O_2} less than 40 mm Hg!

At the opposite extreme is the observation that patients with hypertension, even of a severe degree, usually have normal cerebral blood flow. The inescapable conclusion is that cerebral vasoconstriction also participates in the generalized vascular phenomenon. While the mechanism of this cerebral vasoconstriction remains unproved, it most assuredly is not due to sympathetic α-adrenoreceptor stimulation. Cerebral vessels are sympathetically innervated but show neither α nor β adrenergic effects. Thus they do not participate in the body-wide vasoconstrictive response to baroreceptor or chemoreceptor mediated sympathetic discharge as in the diving reflex.

Cerebral vessels do exhibit the property of autoregulation, the intrinsic property of regulation flow constancy despite rather wide fluctuation in perfusion pressure. In other words, cerebral vessels resist over- or under-perfusion of the brain (at normal Ca_{O_2}) by appropriate adjustment of vessel bore. The mechanism of this effect remains obscure but its importance in cerebral blood flow regulation under conditions ranging from hypoxemia to hypertension should be obvious.

Thus cerebral vessels can exhibit a wide latitude of vasomotor responses to suit particular circumstances, in each case the object of which is to preserve brain function. Unconsciousness and attendant postural collapse associated with hypotension itself protects cerebral blood flow by removing the gravitational disadvantage of head-up posture.

Another feature of cerebral circulation is the limited permeability of capillary endothelium. In marked contrast with the fenestrated, highly permeable type of endothelium found in renal glomerular capillary loops, hepatic and other sinusoids and in the choroid plexus, cerebral capillary endothelium is of the continuous type where intercellular junctions are tightly joined with a minimum of gaps or clefts. In addition, the basement membrane seems to be thicker than usual. The point of this is that while diffusible substances, especially respiratory gases and water, traverse capillary walls without difficulty, other substances do so with substantially greater delay than in other capillary beds. The term blood-brain barrier is used to describe this unusual relative impermeability. Presumably its purpose is to protect brain cells from sudden alterations of its milieu. It should be noted, however, that the degree of impermeability is not uniform in all parts of the brain nor is it immune to alteration by disease processes.

CORONARY CIRCULATION

Special features of the coronary circulation include systolic extravascular compression, low oxygen transport reserve, autoregulation, strong link to metabolic activity and cardiac inotropy and unimpressive response to α-adrenergic stimulation.

Major coronary arterial branches lie on the epicardial surface along their entire path giving off branches at right angles that penetrate the myocardium branching further as they do so. These intramyocardial arteries are so intimately embedded in layers of myocardium that they are throttled by high left ventricular systolic intramyocardial tension. Such extravascular compression also squeezes blood from intramyocardial capillaries and veins. During the enusing diastole, flow into this empty segment is enhanced. This effect, especially the arterial component, is virtually absent in the right ventricular myocardium. Thus flow velocity records from the left and right main coronary arteries are different, the left showing markedly diminished systolic flow and predominating diastolic flow, whereas in the right a normal pattern is seen where systolic flow predominates. The significance of this phenomenon lies in the fact that diastolic pressure gradient is the major determinant of left coronary flow and anything that diminishes aortic diastolic pressure tends to compromise it. Also, since the higher left ventricular wall tension the greater the compressive effect, left ventricular hypertension and dilatation exaggerate it because of the Laplace relation. Left ventricular outflow obstruction is particularly damaging in this regard because it creates high myocardial wall tension while simultaneously producing a discrepancy between left ventricular and aortic systolic pressures.

At rest coronary blood flow in man accounts for about 5% of the cardiac output, but the P_{O_2} of coronary venous blood is quite low, perhaps only a third of that of the average of all other venous effluents. This should not be surprising considering that the heart itself is not resting. On the other hand, the value means that even when producing minimal energy output, myocardial P_{O_2} is at a low level. This reflects the fact that relative to its level of O_2 consumption ($M\dot{V}_{O_2}$), myocardial blood flow is low. Another way to put this is that whereas the body at rest receives an O_2 supply three times what it is actually consuming (this is mainly accounted for by high renal blood flow), the heart only receives a supply in excess of use of perhaps 50–100%.

The significance of this situation should be obvious. Greater total energy output of the heart ($\int T dt + \int P dv + \frac{1}{2} mv^2$) to meet greater demands associated with activity of the organism can be satisfied only by quantitatively appropriate flow increases (i.e., 1:1 with respect to $M\dot{V}_{O_2}$). To the extent this fails to occur, myocardial P_{O_2} will fall. Since coronary perfusion pressure gradient is fixed to the extent arterial blood pressure is regulated by baroreceptors, clearly coronary flow changes are directly dependent upon vascular conductance changes ($\dot{Q} = K g$ or $\dot{Q} = K r^4$).

Given the foregoing equation, the capacity for coronary vasomotion, especially active dilatation, is prodigious. When cardiac energy demands are minimal (organism at rest), coronary vasomotor tone is high; so much so that there is no wasted myocardial perfusion—for practical purposes most of the O_2 delivered is utilized. That vasoconstriction is not maximal, however, can be gleaned from the fact that to the extent $M\dot{V}_{O_2}$ is lowered (artifically such as by BP lowering drugs, reducing temperature, heart rate, or contractility or physiologically, as occurs in estivation or hibernation) coronary vessels constrict even further. During artificial coronary perfusion, increasing flow above a physiologic level results in coronary vasoconstriction and a higher perfusion pressure. In other words, the heart resists accepting more flow than it needs to perform a certain level of work. This is why during open heart surgery when the heart is potassium-arrested (cardioplegia) its O_2 and blood flow requirements are minimal and especially so when hypothermia (cooling) is added as well. Under this circumstance of minimal $M\dot{V}_{O_2}$, coronary vasoconstriction is maximal.

When $M\dot{V}_{O_2}$ is increased by any combination of increased heart rate, temperature, tension generation, external PV and kinetic work, and contractility, coronary vasodilatation occurs. All these effects occur during effort and the cardiac component of chronic physical conditioning obviously involves maximizing them. The fundamental stimulus for dilation to keep pace with $M\dot{V}_{O_2}$ is tissue hypoxia. Thus, even without increasing $M\dot{V}_{O_2}$, coronary vasodilation can be demonstrated by perfusing the coronaries with hypoxemic blood (with P_{CO_2}, pH, and temperature held constant). The lower Ca_{O_2}, the more coronary flow increases up to maximal levels that may be prodigious. Berne has proposed that the link between $M\dot{V}_{O_2}$ (hence tissue P_{O_2}) and coronary vasomotion is mediated by adenosine, a vasoactive adenine nucleotide, rather than the direct effect of P_{O_2}.

Given a fixed external work load (i.e., fixed pressure, stroke volume, and heart rate) but changing the inotropic state of the heart by cardiac sympathetic nerve stimulation or infusion of β-adrenoreceptor stimulating agents (epinephrine or isoproterenol) causes $M\dot{V}_{O_2}$ to increase proportional to that of inotropic state. In this situation coronary vessels dilate and blood flow increases, consistent with the interpretation that it is $M\dot{V}_{O_2}$ and not external work that controls vasomotion. The significance of this is that in circumstances where increments in blood flow may be precluded, such as in severe coronary vascular obstruction by atherosclerosis, sympathetic stimulation can be downright deleterious in calling for blood flow increments that cannot be delivered. At times this is so much so that it becomes a mechanism for myocardial ischemia and even infarction (ischemic tissue death).

Inotropy induced vasodilatation has two possible components. The first is obligatory and has already been discussed; that tied to increased MV_{O_2}. Persumably this type occurs in inotropic enhancement not sympathetically mediated, such as associated with the force frequency and Anrep effects. The second type is that mediated by coronary vascular β-adrenoreceptor stimulation. The notion here is that cardiac sympathetic nerve stimulation or administration of epinephrine or isoproterenol produce not only myocardial inotropic effects which lead to vasodilatation, they have a primary vascular effect as well. The difficulty of separating the two components of vasodilatation should be obvious. Nonetheless, to the extent that the notion is applicable, it represents another example of redundancy nature has devised when something important is at stake.

A corollary of the potent effects of β-adrenoreceptor stimulation is the weakness of α-adrenergic coronary vasoconstriction. There has been much controversy concerning whether it occurs; reflecting, no doubt, the difficulty of separating diametrically opposite effects from a common stimulus, especially when one is negligible. Thus, the coronary circulation is more like cerebral circulation with regard to its insensitivity to sympathetic α-adrenergic vasoconstriction. The teleologic sense of such unresponsiveness in these vascular beds is not difficult to glean, especially in light of the diving reflex or chemoreceptor-mediated sympathetic discharge, situations in which preserving the brain and heart is paramount. Finally, it should be noted that phylogenetically the coronary vessels had their origin in the branchial vessels. Therefore, they are related more to gill and pulmonary vessels than to systemic vessels. It is well known that both gill and pulmonary vessels vasodilate rather than constrict in response to sympathetic mediators so it is really not surprising that the coronaries share this effect.

It has long been suspected that coronary artery constriction (spasm) might account for clinical episodes of myocardial ischemia (this often elicits a characteristic form of chest pain that is termed angina pectoris). There was no great insight as to the specific locus of such an effect, much less its mechanism, except that electrocardiographic evidence suggested a major coronary artery branch. The advent of radiographic angiography (still or motion x-ray films of shadows of blood vessels filled—injected—with radiopaque dyes) has demonstrated conclusively that major coronary branches do exhibit segmental narrowing in response to certain stimuli and that this may indeed be a mechanism for myocardial ischemia in certain patients. The mechanism of this effect is unknown and it accounts for only a small percentage of patients suffering angina pectoris. In the overwhelming majority, vascular obstruction results from atherosclerosis.

RENAL CIRCULATION

Special features of the renal circulation relate to the organ's excretory function. Excluding the lung and chemoreceptors, the kidneys receive the highest blood flow on a unit weight basis of any tissue in the body (400 ml/min/100 g), accounting for 20% of the resting cardiac output. It may be inferred from the high energy cost that this represents that nature has assigned a high priority to the survival value of renal blood flow.

Water enters the body only from the gastrointestinal tract but it can leave by way of skin, lungs, bowel, and kidney. All these exit pathways participate in regulation of water balance to some extent depending on particular circumstances (species, temperature, humidity, etc.), but in most mammalian species, it is on the kidneys that this function depends primarily.

The high renal blood flow is essential for the formation of an adequate volume of glomerular filtrate. Normally, 20% of renal plasma flow (or 10% of renal blood flow) begins the journey out the excretory system as glomerular filtrate. The formation of this ultrafiltrate is a purely physical phenomenon. The blood, in effect, is sieved in the glomerular capillaries. This is accomplished by a high glomerular capillary pressure, roughly 50–60 mm Hg. The mechanisms for such a high pressure are twofold: There are two competing avenues for egress of fluid entering the glomerular capillaries, one is the efferent arteriole and the other is the excretory channel beginning in Bowman's capsule. Fluid flow in the two paths will be distributed according to their relative hemodynamic resistances. In each path these will be the sum of all series resistances including viscosity, vessel bore, fluid movement through tubule walls, etc. The total conductance of these parallel paths (the sum of the individual conductances) is quite low (high resistance) compared to the outflow resistance of other capillary beds, for this is how glomerular capillary filtration pressure is kept high. The conductance of the efferent arteriole path must be the greater of the two since 90% of the fluid (counting red blood cells as fluid volume) takes this route. Of the 10% that is filtered (roughly 120 ml/min), 99% returns to the blood, most of this across the proximal convoluted tubule epithelium. The balance, 1–2 ml/min, is excreted as urine. Nephrologic dogma has it that proximal tubular reabsorption is owing to obligatory water transport associated with active sodium pumping from lumen to peritubular capillary. Why such a mechanism is invoked when it could be accomplished by hemodynamic forces has always escaped me. My faith in nature is offended by such a biologic energy waste. I have had the biased and totally undocumented hypothesis that isosmotic proximal tubular reabsorption of water and solute is owing to the high outflow resistance offered by the long loop of Henle. Since the length of these loops varies depending on whether the nephrons are cortical, medullary or anything in between, the tendency for such "reabsorption" also would be variable. This mechanism would explain why birds and certain desert rodents have only nephrons with Henle loops of such exaggerated length. They have a particular need to conserve water. This hemodynamic reabsorption force (i.e., high proximal tubule pressure) is aided and abetted by the enhanced (by 20%) plasma osmotic and lower hydrostatic pressure in the peritubular capillaries owing to loss of water in the glomerular capillaries and efferent arteriolar resistance, respectively (the relationship between plasma protein concentration and osmotic pressure is curvilinear, the latter increasing significantly at higher protein concentration).

The dribble of fluid reaching the distal tubules is processed still further by the effects of ADH and aldosterone on distal tubule epithelium with respect to additional water reabsorption and exchange of potassium for hydrogen and sodium, respectively.

The important point is that urine formation, at least in its early stages (i.e., glomerular filtration), depends on hemodynamic considerations as much as on cellular secretive processes to effect water balance. The effectiveness of this process is compromised by a reduction in glomerular filtration pressure. A drop in blood pressure would tend to have such an effect, but the kidney autoregulates blood flow; that is, it vasodilates when pressure falls. On the other hand, hypotension elicits baroreflex sympathetic discharge and renal arterioles (presumably afferent and efferent ones) are highly sensitive to α-adrenergic stimulation unlike those in the cerebral and coronary circulations. Thus the net effect depends on which effect predominates. The generalization can be made, however, that in times of circulatory stress such as hypotension, exercise or congestive heart failure, renal excretory function is diminished. Thus, autoregulation seems to be overridden by α-adreneregic vasoconstriction, an effect that provides the possibility of temporary redistribution of normally substantial renal blood flow.

SKIN CIRCULATION

The special feature of the blood supply to skin has to do with temperature regulation.

The mass of skin (3–4 kg) is second only to that of skeletal muscle. The surface area of skin in most adult humans (excluding dwarfs and pygmies) is approximately 1.2–2.4 sq m, and in the resting state at comfortable ambient temperature receives about 10% of the cardiac output. The inherent oxygen requirement of the skin, however, is quite low. It is because skin circulation in humans is the major factor in maintenance of a constant body temperature that gives it special significance.

Heat is a byproduct of exothermic chemical reactions. The rate at which some such reactions occur, in turn, is determined by the temperature of the environment in which they take place. What we call metabolism, metabolic rate or oxygen consumption, therefore, is a measure of this rate. In poikilothermic species this rate waxes and wanes with the external environmental temperature because they do not possess a mechanism for regulating body temperature independent of ambient temperature. Thus, as their body temperature fluctuates with environmental temperature, so too does metabolism. To call such species cold blooded speaks only half the truth, for under certain conditions their blood actually may be warmer than ours. Poikilotherms do have an upper temperature limit, however, because proteins are denatured at high temperatures. Obviously they have developed methods to avoid exposure to such high temperatures.

Homeothermic species, on the other hand, are characterized by a relatively high metabolic rate and body temperature, at least most of the time. Those species that estivate or hibernate have the unusual ability to enter a state of dormancy characterized by marked lowering of metabolism and temperature, the latter essentially to that of the

environment (contrary to popular belief bears are not true hibernators).

Maintenance of body temperature at whatever level represents the
balance between total heat production and loss. If the former is variable, then so must the latter if a regulated temperature is to be
achieved. Resting metabolism and body temperature are not uniform
among mammals being roughly inversely porportional to body mass.
Considering the wide variability in environmental conditions which
various species choose as their natural habitat, it should be apparent
that equally variable heat conserving and losing mechanism must exist
in nature. Skin serves a key role in these processes in man, the only
terrestrial mammal whose integument has been denuded, because
heat loss is determined by skin blood flow, aided and abetted by
perspiration. (Perspiration is quite variable among mammals; for example, dogs do not—they lose heat by panting—whereas camels do
sweat).

There are several determinants of skin blood flow. The most obvious is the level of metabolic activity of the organism, for this is
directly proportional to heat production. Thus when body metabolism (and heat production) is at a minimum level, such as during
sleep, skin blood flow also is near the minimal level. As metabolism
increases with activity, so too must skin blood flow if body temperature is to remain constant. Actually, body temperature does fluctuate
a matter of a few degrees during the day so the activity to skin blood
flow balance is not perfect.

Environmental temperature is another determinant of skin blood
flow that is independent of activity. Skin blood flow is reduced in cold
(up to a point) and increased in hot environments for rather obvious
reasons. In the first instance heat conservation is the goal whereas in
the second it is to enhance heat loss. If the ambient temperature is
higher than that of the body (i.e., greater than 99° F), there is a
predictable problem in achieving the latter goal, for the gradient of
temperature is in the wrong direction for heat removal.

Nature has dealt with this problem effectively (although civilized
man has confounded her purposes by wearing clothing). Man is
armed with sweat glands over most of the skin surface. Sweat is a
hypotonic salt solution secreted by the cells of these glands, but having its origin in the blood. The evaporation of the water in sweat has

a caloric equivalent of 0.58 kcal/ml. Thus, the amount of heat loss that can be accomplished by sweating relates to the volume of sweat and the rate of its evaporation. Under maximal conditions this is of the order of 1.5 liters/hour, which if all evaporated results in removal of some 900 kcal of heat/hr. Basal heat production is only 70 kcal/hr and roughly a fourth of this is removed by cutaneous evaporation. Skin circulation, therefore, serves the dual role of bringing heat to the surface of the body where it gains access to the environment for removal by direct radiation, conduction, convection or evaporation and of providing the fluid for the last process. Sweat by itself is ineffective in accomplishing heat loss for if it is unaccompanied by the vascular component (vasodilatation) all that results is a cold clammy skin. This is a common situation in patients in shock, even those who may have fever. It must be the case, therefore, that there comes a time/situation when even temperature control mechanisms are overridden by a higher priority such as maintaining blood pressure.

Ordinarily, however, temperature control has a high priority in regulation of skin blood flow; the direct measure of this being the extent to which body temperature remains constant, or nearly so, despite wide fluctuation in activity level and environments in which these are undertaken. How then is skin blood flow regulated in the complex situations in which man purposely or inadvertently gets or finds himself (such as swimming the cold English channel, running a marathon or fighting a war on a hot humid day, or falling unconscious in a drunken stupor in a cold environment).

Arterial supply to the skin is of two types, the ordinary or nutritional system ending in capillaries and the arteriovenous shunt pathways that bypass capillaries. The latter are especially abundant in the fingers, more so at the ends. The bore of these anastomotic channels are under potent smooth muscle control to the extent they may be completely closed (nutritional flow only) or open to varying degrees allowing for marked variation in flow up to a maximum approaching that of myocardial (100 ml/min/100 g)! Where shunts are not present, the flow range is more restricted; perhaps 1 ml/min/100 g to 35 ml/min/100 g in the fully dilated state. Thus both systems of vessels have remarkable potential for flow regulation by vasomotor activity.

Skin blood flow virtually comes to a standstill when a low concentration either epinephrine or norepinephrine is injected intraarterially. Sympathectomy or sympathetic blockade, on the other hand, results in marked skin vasodilatation. Thus, skin circulation is perhaps the best example of a circulation that is under the dominant regulation of the sympathetic nervous system. As with vagal heart rate control, skin sympathetic vasoconstriction can be diminished (vasodilatation) or enhanced further from some set point level. The environmental temperature-skin blood flow relationship is mediated by the direct local effect of temperature on vascular smooth muscle and by the effect of a change in core temperature on skin sympathetic vasomotor tone. The direction and magnitude of the latter response would be such as to maintain constancy of body temperature (i.e., negative feedback). The metabolic rate-skin blood flow relationship is also mediated by the effect of core temperature changes on skin sympathetic vasoconstrictor tone. Thus, there is a central temperature receptor that functions much like the baroreceptors, the effector output of which is the level of α-adrenergic vasoconstrictor tone to skin blood vessels. This is accompanied by a sympathetic (cholinergic) outflow to the sweat glands in the instance of an increase in core temperature. The central thermoregulatory mechanism is in the hypothalamus and there are separate centers for achieving heat conservation and loss. Were this not the case it would be difficult to imagine how heat loss could be accomplished since it involves simultaneously increasing sympathetic outflow to sweat glands while diminishing sympathetic skin vasomotor tone. As in the case of the vagal cardiac inhibitory center and the sympathetic vasomotor center, the hypothalamic thermoregulatory centers are reciprocally innervated such that the stimulation of one inhibits the other. The heat conservation center not only produces skin vasoconstriction to reduce heat loss, it induces involuntary generalized repetitive skeletal muscle contractions (i.e., shivering), which generates heat, the two effects combining to maintain body temperature. The sympathetic outflow to skin vessels from the heat loss center must be distinct from sympathetic control of their vascular beds under ordinary circumstances because cutaneous circulation is exempted from participation in baroreflex responses. However, in extreme situations such as severe exertion, shock and advanced heart failure, even the thermoregulatory mechanism may be overridden and vasoconstriction prevail.

Other aspects of cutaneous circulation and its regulation are beyond the scope of this presentation. These include peripheral thermoreceptors, vasodilator sympathetic nerves, local axon reflex, effect of bradykinin or other released vasoactive substances (by sweat glands?), and quantitative and possibly qualitative differences in response of skin of different body parts.

SPLANCHNIC CIRCULATION

The special feature of the splanchnic circulation relates to the portal circulation that gives rise to dual hepatic circulation that comprises about a quarter of the resting cardiac output.

The arterial supply to the gut, mesentery, spleen, pancreas, and liver is arranged in parallel with that to all other organs/tissues. The venous effluent of the first four, however, combine to form the portal drainage into the liver sinusoids, where it is joined by hepatic arterial supply to emerge as hepatic venous effluent into the inferior vena cava. This anatomical relationship serves the physiologic purpose of direct delivery of undiluted mesenteric venous blood, laden with the products of intestinal absorption, to the liver for processing. Hemodynamically, it means that the liver sinusoids are arranged in series with the capillary beds of the gut, pancreas and mesentery and the sinusoids of the spleen.

Capillary dynamics of the gastrointestinal circulation probably do not differ drastically from that in other systemic beds even though capillaries of the mucosal surface expose a large surface area to what basically is the outside world. The determinants of water absorption from the gastrointestinal contents presumably are the same ones that operate in all other capillary beds, the balance between capillary pressure (filtration) and plasma osmotic pressure (reabsorption). These forces normally are very nearly balanced. Arteriolar constriction would tend to enhance water absorption as capillary hydrostatic pressure would decline. Sympathetic α-adrenergic vasoconstriction, ADH (pitressin), or angiotensin II all could produce this effect. Vasodilatation would tend to produce the opposite effect, loss of fluid into the bowel. Since splenic and mesenteric veins drain into the portal vein, pressure in the latter obviously has a lot to do with venous pressure effects on intestinal and splenic capillary dynamics. That is to say, increased portal vein pressure would tend to produce intestinal edema and loss of water into the gut.

Determinants of portal vein pressure include the anatomy of reversed branching (coalescence of venous tributaries), mesenteric blood flow rate, and hepatic sinusoidal and venous resistances.

Portal vein blood flow is probably maximal following meals and less at most other times, but the variation is not great. Because portal vein pressure normally is approximately 10 mm Hg, it is clear that hepatic sinusoidal and venous resistances are very low considering a flow as high as something over 1 liter/min. At this level of flow, portal vein blood is still about 85% saturated with oxygen. It is clear, therefore, that the gut is relatively highly perfused, owing, no doubt, to the fact that the same flow also provides O_2 for the liver. Hepatic venous saturation is 65–70%, about the same as the body average. Thus, of oxygen supplied by mesenteric and splenic arterial circulation, two-thirds is removed by the liver and one-third by the gut and spleen. Of total hepatic blood flow, roughly 70–80% is provided by portal vein flow and the balance by hepatic artery. Hepatic arterial O_2 supply constitutes about 30–40% of the total hepatic oxygen consumption.

The significance of this unusual circulatory arrangement is that it is vulnerable to a variety of disease processes which produce obstructions at different sites in the portohepatic system. Most common among these is chronic cirrhosis, fibrous scarring, of the liver, secondary to chronic malnutrition or toxic or inflammatory liver damage such as by chronic alcoholism. Intrahepatic scarring obstructs sinusoidal-portal venous circulation leading to portal venous hypertension. Portal hypertension produces congestion and edema of the gut, mesentery and spleen, ascites (accumulation of fluid in the peritoneal cavity) and esophageal and hemorrhoidal varices (dilated or varicose esophageal and hemorrhoidal veins). Such varices result from the fact that esophagogastric and hemorrhoidal veins represent two of the sites for collateral portal venous drainage, other sites include retroperitoneal tissues and the falciform ligament. Portal hypertension is also caused by prehepatic obstruction, such as by portal vein thrombosis (clot formation) or schistosoma (trematode parasite) infestation. Posthepatic obstruction is most commonly caused by chronic congestive heart failure (i.e., high-venous pressure) but may also result from localized hepatic vein or inferior vena cava obstruction such as by cancer. In these situations hepatic congestion occurs in addition to portal hypertension. Normal hepatic sinusoidal dynamics is characterized by low sinusoidal pressure (5–8 mm Hg) and high permeability, which allows free exchange of plasma proteins. This means that effective plasma protein osmotic pressure is reduced to perhaps a third of its normal value. Thus, the liver is vulnerable to congestion and edema by even minor increase in sinusoidal pressure. The liver capsule limits acute distention to a limited extent but does not prevent chronic enlargement of the liver. An enlarged liver becomes palpable on abdominal examination as its inferior edge emerges below the right costal margin, a characteristic finding in chronic congestive heart failure.

UTERINE CIRCULATION

The special features of uterine circulation relate to menses and pregnancy. This presentation will not concern itself with the former which entails cyclic endometrial suicide by strangulation (infarction or ischemic necrosis) resulting from hormonally regulated vasconstriction of the coiled arteries in the uterus. It is of greater hematologic, endocrine and psychologic concern than of circulatory despite menses being misconstrued as a form of blood flow.

The nongravid uterus also is of trivial consequence in circulation physiology since it accounts for only a minute fraction of total body oxygen consumption and blood flow, the latter being less than 50 ml/min in woman. The special demands of pregnancy changes this situation most drastically, as any mother can attest. At term, the mass of uterus (1 kg) plus fetus is approximately 4–5 kg, twice that of the liver.

The requirement to satisfy the circulatory needs of a growing fetus and enlarging uterus may not be as dramatic as those required in severe muscular effort, but it is far more significant in nature's general scheme of things. The chronicity of pregnancy circulatory demands also place them in categories of significant cardiovascular stresses.

It is hardly surprising that nature has provided redundant arterial and venous pathways for uterine nutrition in the form of paired ovarian and uterine vessels, as well as multiple collateral venous anastomoses. This is necessitated not only to insure adequate fetal nutrition but to transport a blood flow that may reach values as high as one liter per minute or more in multiple pregnancies, a 20% increment in resting cardiac output. Burwell has likened this cardiovascular load to that of an arteriovenous fistula. It is without question an example of high-output states. The chronic high blood flow demand is met by modest increase in heart rate with maintained or increased stroke volume. An augmented circulating blood volume is an important mechanism providing the latter. These effects reach a peak about the 30th wk of gestation and begin declining prior to parturition. Since pregnancy also is associated with increased maternal renal blood flow, it is easy to conceive why the pregnant state provides a measure of the competence of the cardiovascular apparatus to withstand stresses that are additive to those of everyday living.

The placenta is the medium for exchange of all substances between maternal and fetal blood. It is estimated that the chorionic villi provides about 15 sq m of diffusion exchange surface for the transport of gases, water, electrolytes, nutrients, heat, hormones, etc. It is hardly surprising that permeability is sufficiently great that the interface constitutes a barrier only to large molecules and formed blood elements. The significance of this permeability characteristic is that many drugs that enter the maternal circulation gain access to the fetal. Small amounts of red blood cells do cross the placental barrier in some pregnancies for this is the mechanism by which a fetus with Rh positive blood type of an Rh negative mother can sometimes lead to the mother developing antibodies against fetal blood. When such antibodies gain access to fetal blood in sufficient amount, they can produce fetal hemolysis (red cell destruction). Fortunately, the chances of this complication are low.

FETAL CIRCULATION

The fetus develops a cardiovascular system very early for the obvious reason that this is essential for growth and development of all tissues to occur. The fetal heart, therefore, provides the energy for blood flow required to maintain a physiologic environment for all fetal cells. The placenta serves the functions of lungs, kidney, gastrointestinal tract and skin until the umbilical cord is clamped or the placenta separates at birth. Thus, the umbilical artery and vein represent the lifeline on which the fetus depends for a physiologic milieu intérieur and of all the myriad of substances that have to be exchanged across

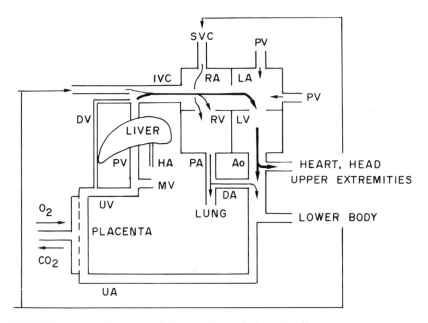

FIGURE 14–1 Diagram of the fetal circulation. Cardiac structures upper right. DA = ductus arteriosus, UA & UV = umbilical artery and vein, respectively, MV = mesenteric veins, PV = portal vein, HA = hepatic artery, DV = ductus venosus. Note shunts through atrial septal defect and ductus arteriosus and fractionation of descending aortic flow to placenta and lower part of body.

the chorionic villi, it is that of oxygen that is paramount. It is true that the fetus is much more tolerant to hypoxia (equivalent to being acclimatized to high altitude dwelling); nonetheless, growth and development are oxygen limited. When the quantitative requirement for O_2 uptake is met, all other substances are adequately exchanged.

The special feature of the fetal circulation, therefore, relates to the anatomic and physiologic mechanisms that provide for distribution of O_2 acquired in the placenta (Figure 14–1).

The fetal liver is the initial recipient of a portion of oxygenated and nutritives-laden blood returning from the placenta. This makes good sense considering the remarkable array and importance of hepatic functions. Umbilical vein blood is about 80% saturated (P_{O_2} 45 mm Hg) and emerges from the liver mixed with fetal portal vein flow as hepatic venous blood with a saturation of approximately 65%. The ductus venosus represents a direct pathway for the remainder of umbilical vein blood to enter the inferior vena cava bypassing the liver. The saturation of the combined effluent is approximately 70% (P_{O2} 35). Most of the inferior caval venous return passes directly to the left atrium through the foramen ovale because of the crista dividens which forms a flap that diverts flow. Another reason that flow through the foramen ovale is the preferred path is right ventricular distensibility less than that of the left (i.e., filling resistance is increased). This is because the collapsed lung constitutes a high resistance path compared to aortic flow. Thus only a fraction of venous return from the cavae, and particularly that from the superior, becomes right ventricular output, and only a fraction of the latter perfuses the lung because the patent ductus arteriosus provides a lower resistance (greater conductance) shunt pathway for the balance of right ventricular output to become a part of aortic blood flow. The two ventricles, therefore, function in parallel rather than in series, a situation somewhat akin to species with single ventricle but parallel inflow and outflow channels. Another benefit that accrues from the two venoarterial shunts is that better oxygenated blood perfuses the brain and heart while their venous effluents, presumably near maximally deoxygenated, is diverted through the patent ductus down the descending aorta where its chances of getting to the placenta for reoxygenation via the umbilical arteries is maximized. The oxyhemoglobin saturation of left ventricular output (a combination of deoxygenated pulmonary venous blood flow and oxygenated foramen ovale shunt flow) is 60–65% whereas that in the descending aorta is 55–60%. Seventy-five percent of descending aortic blood flow (over half of total arterial blood flow) becomes umbilical arterial flow to the placenta. This means that of total fetal cardiac energy consumption and release, roughly half is spent obtaining O_2 and nutrients and eliminating waste and heat and the other other half maintaining a physiologic cell environment, values probably not too different than obtain in the resting adult. However, the fetus, growing and developing completely immersed in water of regulated temperature as it does, the fetal circulation has no gravitational forces to contend with nor need to regulate skin blood flow, elaborate urine or support pulmonary ventilation or sustained exercise.

Birth and the first breath represent the moment of truth for the fetus. Mature ones are up to the task and acquire their full independence with comfortable overlap in switching between placental and pulmonary respiration. The sudden high saturation and P_{O_2} of arterial blood resulting from air breathing serves to close the patent ductus arteriosus while the sudden decrease in pulmonary and increase in systemic vascular resistances leads to reversal of in utero ventricular distensibilities, the right increasing (diminished filling resistance) and left decreasing. Therefore, left atrial pressure rises whereas right atrial falls. The latter is aided and abetted by the fact that inferior vena caval flow drops abruptly by the amount of umbilical vein flow when the cord is clamped (in nature, the umbilical arteries constrict). The flap on the left side of the foramen ovale closes the defect by this reversed pressure gradient causing all venous return to empty into the right ventricle, the adult series connection.

HYPOXEMIA

Hypoxemia refers to reduced oxygen content in arterial blood. This is different than the usual definition, which is that arterial blood oxyhemoglobin saturation is less than complete because of lowered P_{O_2}. Hypoxemia may or may not lead to tissue hypoxia depending on whether blood flow compensation for hypoxemia is adequate. On the other hand, tissues may be rendered hypoxic even though hypoxemia is absent, such as by a reduction in blood flow (i.e., ischemia). The causes of hypoxemia include reduced oxygenation of arterial blood, anemia and defects in hemoglobin O_2 binding. All are common situations that deserve separate consideration (Figure 14–2).

Hypoxemia is a normal condition for people who reside (or fly unpressurized aircraft) over 4000 ft altitude. (It so happens that this is the elevation of Salt Lake City.) At this lower limit ambient P_{O_2} is sufficiently reduced such that arterial P_{O_2} is near the shoulder of the normal oxyhemoglobin dissociation curve where hemoglobin saturation is down to about 93% and P_{O_2} approximately 75 mm Hg. This results in mild, relative (by sea level standards) hyperventilation (P_{CO_2} = 37–38 instead of 40 mm Hg) and, if the stimulus is chronic, polycythemia (percentage of red blood cell volume 47–48, instead of 45) as physiologic compensatory adjustments. Residents of high mountain villages and communities in the Peruvian Andes, the Himalayas, the North American Rockies, the Bolivian plateau, Mexico City, etc. (altitudes 7000–15,000 ft) endure proportionally greater hypoxemia and, accordingly, compensatory effects. Another common

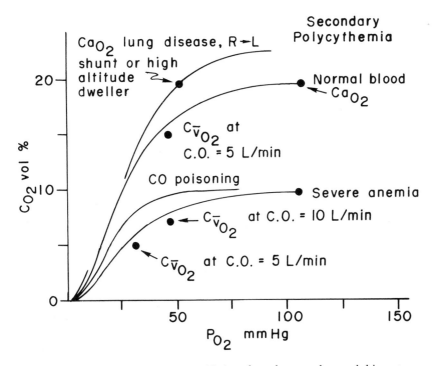

FIGURE 14–2 Oxygen content (C_{O_2}) rather than oxyhemoglobin saturation of blood plotted against P_{O_2} to show effect of hypoxemia, severe anemia, secondary polycythemia and carbon monixide (CO). Hypoxemia without compensation would be any arterial value left of the the normal blood Ca_{O_2} point. Note reduction in mixed venous O_2 content ($C_{\bar{v}O_2}$) in anemia without compensatory increase in cardiac output. Full compensation in O_2 delivery by doubling cardiac output. In polycythemia arterial content is maintained despite reduced P_{O_2} resulting from disorders characterized by hypoxemia.

cause of hypoxemia is pulmonary diseases of diverse etiology and pathophysiologic mechanisms. These include disorders of ventilation, diffusion, and ventilation-perfusion matching. Hypoxemia in these conditions is variable depending on the severity of the process and often is accompanied by elevated rather than depressed P_{CO_2} levels, as is the case with altitude hypoxia. Quite obviously such hypoventilation reflects a failure of hyperventilatory compensation to the hypoxic stimulus. Polycythemia, however, usually is present. A third common cause of hypoxemia is that associated with venoarterial shunting, venous blood getting into the arterial circulation without benefit of ventilation. This is also called venous admixture. It results from a variety of causes too, including congenital cardiac defects, pulmonary disorders (many of the same that cause hypoxemia by other mechanisms), and unusual anatomic venoarterial connections. In these conditions the magnitude of hypoxemia is directly related to the quantity of venous admixture. Polycythemia oftentimes is spectacular and neither hypercapnia nor hypocapnia is present in congenital heart disease with venoarterial shunting because the blood that is ventilated is hyperventilated by an amount sufficient to compensate for that which is not. The most common cause of venous admixture associated with pulmonary disease is perfusion of alveoli or lung segments that are not ventilated because of airway obstruction. Polycythemia, while it is compensatory as far as increasing O_2 content in the face of desaturation, presents a problem as far as increased flow compensation is concerned because it increases blood viscosity markedly at red cell volume percentages in excess of 60%. Some polycythemic patients feel better when their polycythemia is reduced from severe levels by multiple phlebotomy (blood removal).

Anemia undoubtedly is the most common cause of hypoxemia in the world because the disease is common in underdeveloped countries. Most physiologists and physicians do not classify anemia as a form of hypoxemia with valid reason. I don't know that I can justify my doing so considering that the O_2 saturation of hemoglobin in and the P_{O_2} of arterial blood are both normal in anemia. However, because of the deficiency of hemoglobin (remember that each gram of hemoglobin combines with 1.34 ml of O_2), arterial blood O_2 content, Ca_{O_2}, is reduced in direct proprotion to the severity of hemoglobin reduction. Thus, O_2 transport is compromised qualitatively the same way as with desaturation (real hypoxemia) of normal amounts of hemoglobin. The difference is that anemic hypoxemia can be compensated only by an increase in cardiac output whereas that associated with hemoglobin unsaturation stimulates polycythemia, as well as increased flow. When these compensations are quantitatively appropriate, no tissue hypoxia results and this is usually the case under resting conditions. However, the increased O_2 demands associated with exercise, fever, hyperthyroidism, etc., are met with difficulty, inadequately or not at all. When anemia develops gradually, as it usually does, it is remarkable the extent to which flow compensation and acclimation (development of tolerance to low levels of tissue P_{O_2}) compensate in otherwise healthy people. It is not at all uncommon to encounter patients with red cell volume percentages as low as 10–15% with only mild to moderate limitation of sedentary daily activities.

Carbon monoxide (CO) inhalation is another cause of hypoxemia despite normal arterial blood P_{O_2}. In the past, carbon monoxide poisoning was virtually always accidental (poorly ventilated combustion) or suicidal (automobile exhaust) and while these continue, other forms are now recognized. Chronic heavy cigarette smoking or inhalation of heavily polluted (with CO) air can produce mild but significant CO toxicity in some people. Carbon monoxide binds with the iron of heme the same way O_2 does except that the affinity is over 200 times greater. Thus inhalation of very low levels of CO will saturate hemoglobin compared with high O_2 levels required. The other bad feature of carbon monoxide hemoglobin (carboxyhemoglobin) besides that of displacing O_2 is that it shifts the oxyhemoglobin dissociation curve leftward. At normal levels of alveolar P_{O_2} this does nothing to enhance O_2 uptake in the lungs but it markedly diminishes O_2 release in the tissues. This explains why for similar degrees of reduction in arterial blood O_2 content in anemia and CO poisoning, the latter is much more poorly tolerated and compensated. Subclinical chronic CO hypoxemia may be of no great consequence to a normal inactive person living at sea level but it is hardly trivial in patients with ischemic, anemic or other hypoxic diseases, especially if they reside at high altitude. Another consideration worthy of note in this regard is pregnancy and fetal O_2 supply. The latter is marginal enough, especially at altitude, without the difficulty being compounded by both maternal and fetal hemoglobin being rendered useless and less efficient as oxygen carriers. Cigarette smoking should be forbidden for expectant mothers (especially altitude dwellers) unless they agree to live in a hyperbaric oxygen chamber. The latter is highly effective and useful in the treatment of CO poisoning because by increasing P_{O_2} 10- to 20-fold, oxygen affinity for heme is enhanced in its competition with CO.

There is another way that O_2 binding to heme is obviated and that is when the ferrous (Fe^{++}) form of heme iron is converted to the ferric (Fe^{+++}). This form of heme iron is called methemoglobin (ferrihemoglobin) and it may be found in higher than normal ($< 0.1\%$) concentrations associated with certain drugs, especially nitrites. Significant methemoglobinemia is a relatively rare condition.

Cardiac output (CO) augmentation represents the cornerstone of the physiologic response to hypoxemia, for without it tissue hypoxia is virtually inevitable. This is evident from the relationship: tissue P_{O_2} α $Ca_{O_2} - \dot{V}_{O_2}/CO$. That is to say, as Ca_{O_2} falls the only way the ratio $\dot{V}_{O_2}/CO$ can be reduced to maintain tissue P_{O_2} is for $\dot{V}_{O_2}$ to fall, CO to increase, or both. Oxygen consumption may fall when things get very bad, but ordinarily it is on CO increase that the body depends.

What mechanism accounts for increased cardiac output associated with hypoxemia? On the surface of it, one would not expect baroreceptor stimulation and response to be involved on the grounds that by and large these are chronic rather than acute effects, the lack of evidence that blood pressure is reduced in these conditions and the absence of other manifestations of sympathetic stimulation, such as resting tachycardia, on a consistent or uniform basis (some patients with anemia do have it).

Since blood pressure usually is normal in these conditions in the face of elevated cardiac output, clearly peripheral vascular resistance is reduced. This feature characterizes so-called high output states. The mechanism of reduced resistance in these conditions is vasodilatation (due to reduced tissue P_{O_2} relative to metabolic activity or to problems in O_2 utilization) or the presence of arteriovenous shunts or aortic valve leakage. This suggests that reduced peripheral resistance by itself is a mechanism for increased cardiac output. There is evidence to support this notion. Warner showed in dogs that when the muscular vasodilation of exercise was offset by graded artificial occlusion of the aorta, cardiac output increase could be prevented. He concluded that reduced aortic impedance (compliance, resistance, and inductance) is an important determinant of cardiac output response to exercise. There is a currently popular form of therapy for heart failure that hinges on this principle. It is called afterload reduction and consists of parenteral or oral administration of any of a number of vasodilator agents. It provides the benefit of reducing ventricular filling pressures while increasing cardiac output with only minor reduction in blood pressure.

An elevated cardiac output without systematic tachycardia implies stroke volume augmentation. The combination of increased vascular capacity associated with vasodilatation and greater stroke volume suggests that blood volume expansion is a contributory component of the cardiovascular compensation for hypoxemia. Measurements of plasma and red cell volumes in high-altitude residents and sojourners have been made substantiating such a mechanism. Blood volume is also elevated in patients with pulmonary disorders accompanied by hypoxemia. It is important to note, however, that hypoxic pulmonary vasoconstriction occurs in both altitude and lung disease dependent types of hypoxemia leading to chronic right ventricular-pulmonary hypertension. This by itself is a stimulus for enhanced circulating blood volume.

Blood volume also has been found to be increased in severe anemia. Because the erythropoietic (red blood cell forming) system is compromised, such volume augmentation depends on expanded plasma volume. This compounds anemia because of dilution but it provides the advantage of compensatory cardiac output increase that does not depend on sympathetic stimulation. The mechanism of blood volume augmentation in the high output states (hypoxemia, anemia, hyperthyroidism, arteriovenous shunts, thiamin deficiency, pregnancy, and aortic valve regurgitation) is unknown but candidates would include the renin–angiotensin–aldosterone, ADH, and, possibly, chemoreceptor mechanisms.

15
SHOCK

There is no clinical or experimental condition the understanding of which provides clearer insights into circulation physiology in its many ramifications than does shock. Undoubtedly, this is because hardly any circulatory parameter is unaffected by this complex condition.

Shock may be defined as a clinical or experimentally produced syndrome of diverse etiology characterized by acute or subacute deficiency in cardiac output relative to metabolic demand, commonly accompanied by reduction in blood pressure. Ordinarily, oxygen delivery is what is lacking, but rarely other metabolic constituents may be involved such as thiamine or adrenocortical steroids. A low cardiac output by itself does not define the shock state because it is commonly found that low output associated with chronic heart failure is lower than that found in shock. Indeed, it is possible to find normal cardiac outputs in patients with fully developed shock. This usually will be in clinical states associated with elevated demand. Thus, it is the acute nature of the process that circumvents/overwhelms physiologic compensatory mechanisms that seems to be critical in pathogenesis.

Arterial blood pressure usually will be reduced in shock; perhaps invariably so in its terminal phases, but it is not unusual to find (especially when direct measurements are made) normal blood pressure in certain patients or in certain phases of certain types of shock. Because it is possible to find low blood pressure in people not in shock, the absolute level of blood pressure is an unreliable index of the shock state, notwithstanding the ease and relative reliability of its measurement.

Lactic acidemia also occurs in shock; again, perhaps indubitably so in its terminal stages, but here, too, its presence and/or level in a definition of shock lacks specificity and sensitivity in some patients or in some types of shock. Thus, there is no single parameter, the qualitative presence or quantitative value of which unerringly will define shock, particularly in its early stages when correct diagnosis is most critical. The reason for this diagnostic difficulty is the intricate defense (compensatory) mechanisms that nature has evolved to prevent fatality in the animal or person suffering shock. The very cardiovascular oxygen transport reserve that allows higher organisms to deal effectively with the vicissitudes of a sometimes hostile environment are the same mechanisms that make precise quantitative diagnosis (and definition) of shock difficult.

The most important thing that can be said to physicians (or would-be physicians) about shock is that it should be prevented. Why this simple message is so poorly received (or comprehended) is difficult to understand considering that shock represents failure of highly sophisticated, commonly redundant, and usually effective (although not fail-safe) physiologic mechanisms that are designed to protect vital organs according to a well-ordered hierarchy. Nature's attitude concerning such failure in individuals is to say that such hapless victims are expendable—and good riddance if preservation of the species (i.e., by survival of the fittest) is enhanced thereby. In this context the practice of medicine, especially in its aggressive, all-out form, is to defy nature's principle of expendability of weakened individuals, because it has as its prime goal preservation of every individual—whatever the consequences to the species.

Aggressive and, more especially, early intervention are already having an important impact on shock mortality statistics, but the success rates were abysmal to start with, which means there is still a long way to go to achieve unmitigated success. Fundamental to effective dealing with shock is understanding its varied and multifactoral precipitating mechanisms and the cascading or vicious-circle effects that lead to a final common pathway of lethal irreversibility.

Since cardiac output is the product of only two physiologic variables, heart rate and stroke volume, obviously changes in cardiac output are explicable on the basis of alterations of either or both variables in a virtually infinite number of possible combinations. Each has its own determinants that may be affected by the inciting mechanism or by physiologic responses to it. For example, an ectopic or reentrant atrial tachyarrhythmia if sufficiently rapid (especially if it were to occur in a patient with some underlying heart disease who is more predisposed to it), can easily cause such interference with ventricular filling that stroke volume falls to a degree such that cardiac output falls despite the fast heart rate. The tendency for blood pressure to fall resulting therefrom would be sensed by the carotid sinus and aortic arch baroreceptors as requiring a response to counteract the effect. Such a compensatory response includes lessened vagal and

heightened sympathetic cardiac stimulation and sympathetic vasoconstriction. The effect on contractility is appropriate (i.e., increase), but
the chronotropic effect is not, particularly the tendency of decreased
vagal tone to enhance conduction through the AV node. Actually, a
higher degree of vagally mediated AV block would be desirable, especially in atrial tachyarrhythmias such as flutter. Clearly, it is not
enough to know what the heart rate is; it is also important to know
what its mechanism is. Clincial clues are helpful and useful to determine this but an electrocardiographic rhythm record is indispensable.
Similarly, a slow heart rate is totally inappropriate in the context of
a reduced blood pressure. It means either that the rate is slow because
of an abnormal electrical mechanism not subject to vagal control (such
as complete heart block) or there is abnormally strong vagal stimulation of the SA and/or AV nodes (such as in pain or horror-mediated
vagal reaction) causing sinus bradycardia or undesirable physiologic
AV block.

Stroke volume alterations are of only three types: altered ventricular filling, emptying or both. An example of shock due to disordered
cardiac emptying is sudden obstruction of pulmonary vessels as by
embolism (blood clot, air, amniotic fluid, fat, etc.). Keep in mind,
however, that left ventricular filling becomes impaired when right
ventricular emptying is deficient, a circular problem. The physiologic
response to impaired emptying is an attempt to enhance filling of the
poorly emptying ventricle through the Starling mechanism. This occurs automatically: a ventricle that is unable to eject a normal stroke
volume has a higher residual volume and is already set up to have
greater filling on the subsequent beat. This is aided and abetted by
right atrial volume increases by venoconstriction and right atrial contractility enhancement by the Frank–Starling mechanism. Superimposed on these intrinsic mechanisms, the reduction in left ventricular
output and arterial pressure incites baroreflex sympathetic cardiac
chronotropy and inotropy and arteriolar and venous constriction, the
former to maintain arterial pressure and the latter to enhance right
ventricular filling. If this chain of interrelated events proves inadequate, cardiac output, and ultimately blood pressure, will fall and
eventuate in the shock state.

A disorder of cardiac emptying that by itself accounts for more
cardiovascular deaths than all others combined is that associated with
acute myocardial infarction (cardiogenic) shock. If the mass of myo-

cardium suffering ischemic injury by vascular interruption is sufficiently large, a primary defect in left ventricular emptying (i.e., acute left heart failure) occurs. This sets into motion all that was mentioned above, except in this case the need is to enhance filling of the left ventricle and, upstream from it, the left atrium and pulmonary veins and capillaries. The latter creates the potential for an undesirable complication. Left heart filling pressure governs pulmonary capillary pressure which can increase only to the ceiling of plasma oncotic pressure without upsetting the Starling capillary equilibrium that maintains alveolar walls and spaces in a relatively dry state. Acute pulmonary edema (water-congested alveolar walls and spaces) is deleterious because it interferes with gas diffusion, especially of oxygen, leading to arterial blood hypoxemia being superimposed on the ischemic myocardial defect. Uninjured viable myocardium is subjected to increased workload because of the absolute reduction in functional myocardium and the effect of a distended ventricular chamber (Laplace effect) having to generate greater wall tension to develop the same intracavitary pressure. Myocardial oxygen consumption, accordingly, is increased by dilatation. Myocardial injury, if it involves the pacemaker or conducting tissue, often leads to confounding primary rate and/or rhythm disturbances. Occasionally myocardial infarction is accompanied by inappropriate vagal hyperactivity (chemoreceptor mediated?), which causes cardiac slowing by pacemaker suppression, AV block, or both. Hypervagotonia also abrogates peripheral venoconstriction mechanisms designed to enhance venous return. Such a response is reminiscent of the diving and play dead reflex in lower animals, survival value of which is to reduce oxygen consumption to a bare minimum in an attempt to protect the brain. It is hardly surprising that the interaction of the previously mentioned effects commonly results in the shock state.

There are many causes of peripherally mediated disorders of cardiac filling. Hemorrhage, internal or external, spontaneous or traumatic, is the most common and dramatic prototype. Blood that leaves the vascular space, whether from arteries or veins, is subtracted from venous return. Thus, as long as bleeding or other fluid sequestration persists there is a discrepancy between cardiac output and venous return, both gradually declining to the point where the same reflexes previously outlined are provoked. If bleeding occurs internally and is not brisk, these compensatory mechanisms usually will temporarily maintain blood pressure at satisfactory levels (not to mention the propensity to bleed) and the hemorrhage may go unsuspected until the bottom drops out (i.e., shock develops). Pathophysiology similar to hemorrhage occurs in severe diarrhea (e.g., cholera) or in extensive burns. In the former, water and salt are lost and in the latter, plasma.

Venous return also diminishes when vascular capacity suddenly expands without concomitant increase in blood volume. Blood that pools in (i.e., occupies) the extra space is unavailable for cardiac filling, tantamount, therefore, to being lost as in hemorrhage. Usually intravascular pooling occurs as a consequence of the presence of elevated levels of potent vasodilator substances, of which there is a long and varied list. Impaired venomotor tone produces venous pooling while diminished arteriolar and precapillary sphincter tone lowers arterial blood pressure. When veins and arteries are under the influence of potent vasodilators, their capacity to respond to heightened sympathetic stimulation presumably is blunted. Thus, compensatory neuroreflex mechanisms are rendered less effective. This type of pathophysiology is thought to occur in anaphylaxis, endotoxemia and possibly traumatic shock. In canine endotoxin-induced shock, hepatic vein sphincters constrict and pooling occurs in the splanchnic circulation. In head-up tilt table shock, pooling takes place in the lower extremities.

Widespread and sudden (or subacute) reductions in blood flow lead to characteristic alterations in organ function that are absent when equal or even greater reductions in cardiac output occur gradually as a consequence of chronic heart failure. Brain hypoperfusion results in altered sensorium that varies from confusion, agitation, or semiconsciousness to frank coma. Renal function is impaired as a consequence of reduced blood flow and glomerular filtration leading to oliguria or anuria (reduced or absent urine formation) and azotemia (retention of nitrogenous wastes). Maximal skin vasoconstriction produces a cold, pallid/cyanotic, clammy skin that does not function normally in temperature regulation in patients with fever. Muscle and splanchnic beds are also vasoconstricted (except in vasodilatory shock) as blood is shunted to heart and brain. Ultimately even coronary blood flow suffers and, if it is sufficiently severe, myocardial performance may become depressed because of ischemia. In myocardial infarction, such secondary cardiac insult is heaped on a primarily damaged organ.

Inadequate perfusion and a falling blood pressure also set into motion neurohumoral mechanisms to conserve water and reconstitute circulating blood volume. The ADH and renin–angiotensin–aldosterone mechanisms not only retain water, which by itself helps ameliorate falling venous return, cardiac output, and blood pressure, they have primary pressor (blood pressure supporting) activity as well. The presumed rationale for the sum total of all pressor responses, the latter, as well as sympathetic, and catecholamine-mediated vasoconstriction, is to maintain blood pressure so that brain flow will not be compromised, whatever the deprivation of other vascular beds. Nature decided in the scheme of things that an animal without a brain is not worth saving.

When blood pressure falls to low levels in shock, it is safe to say that the process is far advanced. The clinical evidence for this is that mortality rate usually is high when this stage is reached no matter what treatment is instituted. That this is so should come as no surprise to anyone who understands circulation physiology. Not unexpectedly, the longer blood pressure remains low, the worse prognosis is. Thus, therapeutic interventions in shock are more likely to be successful if they are applied early in the course, preferably before blood pressure falls. Unthwarted, cascading events tend to set up a vicious cycle which culminates in sufficient tissue injury such that cell membranes become leaky, subcellular lysozomes are disrupted and their hydrolytic enzymatic contents discharged into interstitial fluid and circulation where they degrade protein indiscriminately. Vasodilator substances are released and vascular endothelium injured. This is the final common pathway of destruction from which there is no return. That the whole process is preventable or, at least, manageable in its early stages in a significant percentage of cases makes this outcome tragic indeed. On the other hand, there are insults in the different categories that are so massive at initiation that no amount of therapy, however vigorous or early, will interdict a lethal outcome.

16
CONGESTIVE HEART FAILURE

Congestive heart failure is a clinical syndrome of diverse etiology characterized by cardiac output inadequate to meet body demand, especially when the latter is increased, such as during exercise or activity, accompanied by abnormal but variable fluid accumulation. The absolute level of cardiac output is not critical for it may be perfectly normal; indeed, it is even characteristically elevated in certain types of heart failure. Whereas the resting cardiac output may be normal, especially during the early stages of heart failure, during exercise it is distinctly reduced from that expected and appropriate. The important point is that, unlike the normal heart, the failing heart is unable to maintain a physiologic cellular environment under all reasonable conditions of demand. Qualitatively, fluid retention is usually present but quantitatively it is quite variable. In the late stages of untreated heart failure, cardiac output reduction and evidence of congestion are impressive. The term dropsy was used in earlier days to denote fluid accumulation in the tissues.

The syndrome develops slowly, usually over a period of a few to several weeks, months, or years. Indeed, it is the chronicity of its development that separates heart failure from shock, both representing inadequate flow conditions of diverse etiology. The same mechanisms may operate in both, but the acuteness of the insult to cardiovascular function precludes edema formation in shock.

Disorders of practically every component of the heart including the pericardium can lead to congestive heart failure. Obviously pathogenesis differs depending on which structure is affected primarily and whether it is in the left or right heart, but the final outcome often is remarkably uniform. This should not be surprising considering that the body has only so many ways to respond to cardiac dysfunction.

The normal heart and especially the conditioned heart (physiologic hypertrophy) does not need to resort to the Frank–Starling energy augmenting mechanism to accommodate ordinary activities that are of limited duration. By using sympathetically mediated heart rate and contractility augmentation (superimposed on the force–frequency and Anrep effects), temporary demands for increased cardiac output can be met without greater diastolic filling. In fact, heart size probably diminishes somewhat rather than increases during upright exercise. Thus, the normal heart functions on a range of ventricular function curves among which it shifts from point to point, moment by moment, maintaining its energy output appropriate to the magnitude of demand. During sleep (particularly so during estivation or hibernation) it is at the minimum point on the minimum (most rightward in the external work–end-diastolic condition relationship) curve. When sympathetically mediated effects are inadequate to provide the cardiac component of chronic and/or repetitive high demands (such as with vigorous training for competitive athletics), the heart hypertrophies. Hypertrophy has the effect of expanding the leftward range of curves which the heart can use to accommodate maximum demands. The combination, hypertrophy plus inotropy, is what produces the cardiovascular component of record-setting maximal athletic performances involving endurance.

A quantitative definition of heart failure, therefore, must include the aspect of diminished capacity to respond to situations of heightened demand. In other words, in the early stages of heart failure it is important to know not so much what the Frank–Starling relationship is at rest, it is whether a progressive loss of curves to the left has occurred that narrows the range of curves to which the heart can shift in response to stress. The failing heart, too, hypertrophies in an attempt to maintain its range of options, but as the disease progresses or ischemia limits hypertrophy (see the following), the range narrows, regardless. Somewhere along the way, probably concurrently, the failing heart resorts to (falls back on) the Frank–Starling mechanism to achieve energy enhancement to meet demands. The cost for utilizing this mechanism is not inconsequential. First, as far as the heart itself is concerned, failure and dilatation mean greater tension generation to produce the same cavitary systolic pressure because of the Laplace relationship, $T = Pr$, and the complex relation of volume to radius, $r = k\sqrt[n]{V}$. This translates to higher myocardial O_2 consumption (i.e., reduced cardiac efficiency—the machine uses more fuel to do the same job). For the body, the need to increase ventricular filling culminates in all those effects collectively known as congestion.

In the earliest stages of heart failure, therefore, depressed cardiac function will be noted only during strenuous activity. To the extent

that patients refrain from such exertion, depressed cardiac performance passes unnoticed. As failure progresses, less-and-less exercise
reveals the encroachment on cardiac reserve. Hemodynamic assessment of cardiac function during this stage shows normal data at rest,
whereas during exercise abnormalities will be found in the relationship between external work (i.e., pressure × volume) and end-diastolic volume or pressure. The possible combinations include: normal
work at elevated filling pressure, decreased work at normal filling
pressure, decreased work at elevated filling pressure. Elevated filling
pressure of the failing left ventricle is transmitted backward into its
reservoir, the left atrium and pulmonary veins and capillaries, producing alveolar wall and possibly alveolar space edema, especially in
the dependent portions of the lung. The clinical manifestation of this
congestion is shortness of breath (dyspnea) associated with exertion.
Right ventricular failure is characterized by systemic congestion but
this usually does not produce peripheral soft tissue edema noticeable
only during exercise unless activity is sustained, such as at the end of
the day. What usually is noted is a decrease in cardiac output, the
clinical manifestation of which is easy fatigability. In global cardiac
failure, combinations of the previous state occur with considerable
individual variability.

Eventually, when encroachment on cardiac reserve is severe, even
the resting curve shifts rightward (and downward). When this happens, hemodynamic abnormalities in ventricular function will be
present even in the resting state, usually consisting of reduced external work, as well as elevated filling pressure. At this late stage, patients
usually are uniformly symptomatic with markedly impaired exercise
tolerance and persistent congestion.

It should be noted that while the ability of the failing ventricle to
perform external (useful) work diminishes progressively, it is not to
say that total ventricular work is diminished. Remember (Chapter 6)
that external work constitutes only a small fraction of total ventricular
contractile energy, the major share relating to tension maintenance
energy ($\int Tdt$). The latter actually increases rather than diminishes
during heart failure, as shown in Figure 16–1, because it is governed
by heart rate, systolic pressure, and ventricular volume. Of these, the
first increases somewhat, the second remains reasonably constant, and
the last characteristically increases as heart failure progresses. Thus,
a more critical definition of heart failure should include the notion

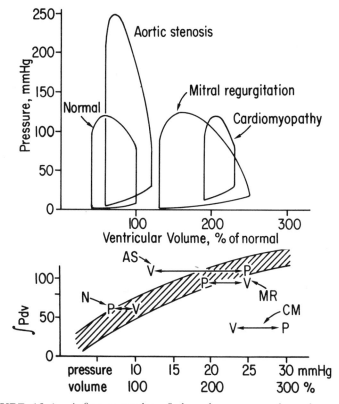

FIGURE 16–1 A few examples of altered pressure volume loops due to various cardiac disease processes and the difficulty of precise definition of heart failure from resting hemodynamics alone (except in the case of cardiomyopathy). The increased pressure work and decreased diastolic ventricular distensibility of aortic stenosis and the increased volume work and increased distensibility of mitral regurgitation are shown. When stroke work loop areas ($\int$ Pdv) are plotted against end-diastolic volume (V) or pressure (P), the Frank–Starling relationship is obtained. The broad band shows approximate normal function from which only cardiomyopathy clearly deviates.

that efficiency is progressively eroded by the declining ratio of useful/total energy (Figure 6–6).

The many kinds of heart disease can be grouped into a few categories as far as the mechanism by which congestive heart failure develops: (1) primary defect in myocardial contractility, (2) defect in myocardial contractility secondary to chronic excessive workload, (3) limitation in cardiac filling, and (4) chronic complete heart block. Some of these are shown in Figure 16–2.

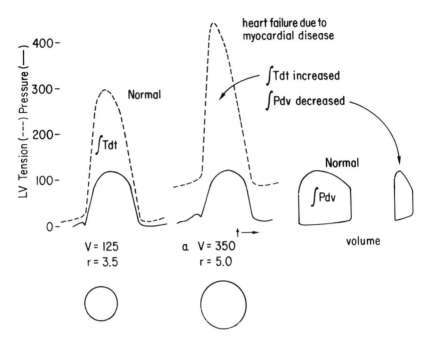

FIGURE 16–2 The energy cost of heart failure (cardiac dilatation and resort to Frank–Starling energy augmenting mechanism). Normal heart is on left of each pair with LV pressure/time (solid line) and tension/time (dotted line) on left and pressure volume loops on right half of figure. In heart failure note elevated end diastolic pressure, end diastolic volume and tension·time energy ($\int$ dt) while external work ($\int$ Pdv) is reduced due to small stroke volume.

In the United States, the most common mechanism for the first category is myocardial ischemia, secondary to obstructive coronary atherosclerosis. Working heart muscle is exquisitely sensitive to oxygen deprivation, quickly manifesting reduced contractility when oxygen supply is lacking. Because obstructive lesions producing ischemia are scattered among the major coronary arteries and their main branches, ischemia usually is patchy rather than global; thus, so too is altered contractility. Therefore, there is a correlation between the mass of myocardium involved in ischemia, its severity, and the manifestations of heart failure. As with any machine, the more that is demanded of it, the more likely it is that depressed performance will be manifest. This is why the earliest signs of heart failure are noted during exertion.

Other forms of failure due to primary depressed contractility include inflammatory (myocarditis), infilitrative (amyloidosis, hemochromatosis) and toxic (alcoholism) disorders and primary myocardiopathies (or cardiomyopathies) in which defects in the contractile machinery of unknown nature occur. In these diffuse myocardial diseases, depressed contractility usually is global and heart failure manifestations severe.

In the second category, congenital or acquired disorders of valves, vessels, septum, etc., place chronic, excessive workloads on the heart, eventuating in failure. Extra work is in the form of ineffectual (wasted) flow, elevated pressure, or both. It is truly remarkable the extent to which the normal heart can adapt itself to such loads. This is particularly so when the burden is congenital or occurs early in life, develops gradually, and there is no interference with concomitant hypertrophy of the coronary circulation to match that of myocardium. Which chamber will bear the brunt of the exaggerated workload depends on the specific lesion. For example, in systemic hypertension, aortic valve stenosis and congenital coarctation of the aorta, the left ventricle is burdened with chronic high pressure load. In aortic and mitral valve regurgitation and patent ductus arteriosus, the left ventricle ejects large stroke volumes, only a portion of which is effective forward cardiac output. In atrial septal defect the right ventricle may eject stroke volumes two- to fivefold larger than the left. In recurrent pulmonary thromboembolism, congenital pulmonic stenosis or idiopathic pulmonary hypertension, right ventricular systolic pressure occasionally exceeds that of the left. As with all diseases there is a spectrum of severity of all these lesions. There are also combinations of them.

The myocardial response to elevated workload is hypertrophy; the same as occurs in skeletal muscle. The type of hypertrophy differs depending on whether the load is excess pressure or stroke volume. In the former, the ventricular wall thickens without dilation (so-called concentric hypertrophy) whereas in the latter the ventricular chamber dilates, as well as increases in mass. Considering the Laplace relationship, $T = Pr$, the advantage of these responses is evident. A chamber having to generate high pressures is at a marked disadvantage if its dilates (large r). Concentric hypertrophy obviates this. A dilated chamber has an advantage in ejecting large stroke volumes for the same extent of sarcomere shortening. Dilation also ameliorates high filling pressure by increasing distensibility. The worst lesions (usually these are combinations) are those that place both a pressure and volume overload on the heart simultaneously.

Hypertrophy is characterized by both increase in the size of myocardial cells and in the total number of myofibrils. More myofibrils per cell means more sarcomeres for force generation. If myocardial hypertrophy is not accompanied by parallel increase in the number of capillaries, average diffusion distance between capillaries and cells increases and average tissue P_{O_2} falls. Thus, a case can be made for relative tissue hypoxia being both the stimulus for myocardial and capillary hypertrophy and also the factor that limits the effectiveness of such compensatory mechanisms. To the extent that myocardial hypertrophy exceeds vascular hypertrophy, the potential exists for cardiac O_2 demand to exceed O_2 supply, a situation commonly referred to as the heart outstripping its blood supply. It is probable, therefore, that the limiting factor in hypertrophy is vascular rather than muscular. If true, the ultimate mechanism for heart failure in category two is the same as that in obstructive coronary vascular disease, namely ischemia. Clinical correlates of such ischemia due to hypertrophy include: (1) ischemic chest pain (angina pectoris) in patients with aortic outflow obstruction in the absence of demonstrable coronary obstruction due to marked left ventricular hypertension and hypertrophy in the face of reduced coronary perfusion pressure gradient. (2) Electrocardiographic so-called ischemic ST segment depression and T wave inversion in diseases characterized by ventricular hypertrophy are indistinguishable from those in patients with obstructive coronary disease. (3) Evidence of compromised ventricular function exaggerated by hypoxemia and during exercise when cardiac O_2 consumption increases.

For each heart so afflicted, the right combination of severity and duration of a particular lesion will eventuate in a situation where compensatory hypertrophy will become inadequate to continue meeting the demands of the excessive (and perhaps increasing) workload. It resorts more and more to the Frank–Starling mechanism to meet exaggerated contraction energy requirements: tension development and external (pressure × volume) work.

The mechanism for increasing ventricular filling volume so that the Frank–Starling mechanism can function involves increased atrial contractility, greater energy expenditure of the opposite ventricle, augmented blood volume, and systemic venoconstriction. As these combine to enhance filling, ventricular diastolic pressure rises according to the ventricle's particular distensibility. Upstream atrail, venous, and capillary pressures are obligated to increase pari passu. The latter is what leads to disordered capillary fluid dynamics and edema formation (i.e., congestion). For the left ventricle, congestion occurs in the lungs. Body tissues become congested when the right ventricle fails. In global myocardial disease, congestion involves both capillary beds. In mitral valve stenosis (narrowing), the obstruction to left ventricular filling and the need to overcome it leads to striking pulmonary congestion while secondary pulmonary arterial hypertension often leads to right heart failure and systemic congestion.

Tricuspid valve stenosis is one of the rare conditions that leads to impressive systemic congestion but does not involve altered ventricular function. As the valve narrows progressively, right atrial and systemic venous pressure has to increase by a factor of the second power in order to maintain flow at the same level. Instead, flow diminishes to ameliorate venous hypertension somewhat. Patients with tricuspid stenosis, therefore, have marked venous hypertension and very low cardiac outputs. Another form of cardiac filling defect that leads to congestive heart failure is constrictive pericarditis. Here the thickened, fibrotic, nondistensible pericardium gradually encroaches on ventricular filling space. The body can't distinguish this effect of progressive reduction in cardiac output from any other form of heart failure and responds accordingly. It aims to increase ventricular filling volume. Unfortunately, all it succeeds in doing is raising filling pressure markedly because the stiff, constricting process precludes a significant volume increment without marked pressure rise. Diastolic pressure in all cardiac chambers is uniformly elevated, being determined not by cardiac distensibility but by that of the extracardiac limiting factor. Thus, congestion occurs in both systemic and pulmonary capillary beds, but fluid retention in the former is far more impressive. The reason for this is that plasma oncotic and capillary hydrostatic pressures in systemic capillaries normally are already at the offsetting (balanced) point whereas in pulmonary capillaries the former is ahead by some 15 mm Hg. The latter provides a cushion accommodating pulmonary capillary hydrostatic pressure rise of this magnitude before pulmonary congestion (alveolar flooding) becomes marked. There is no cushion in the systemic capillaries when venous pressure is persistently elevated.

The kidneys are active participants in the pathogenesis of congestive heart failure because it is through their retention of salt and water that the plasma volume expands. For many years a debate took place between proponents of what were considered to be conflicting hypotheses of the mechanism of congestion associated with heart failure; so-called forward and backward failure theories. In essence, the former held that congestion occurred because of renal salt and water retention secondary to reduced cardiac output, renal plasma flow and glomerular filtration. The main thesis of the latter was that blood backed up behind the failed ventricle. It turns out that the argument was wholly unnecessary. Both sides were describing the same elephant but from feeling different parts. We have sinced learned that the whole salt and water retaining mechanism is much more complex than originally conceived, but that it is involved there no longer remains doubt. There is no doubt also that a failing ventricle (or one that the body thinks is failing such as in cardiac tamponade or constriction) invokes the Frank–Starling mechanism (higher filling volume/pressure) in an effort to enhance its energy output. It is fruitless to debate which is more important, the chicken or the egg; one begets the other and so it is with the failed heart and renal salt and water retention in the pathogenesis of congestion.

The mechanism by which the kidneys retain salt and water in congestive heart failure presumably is no different from that during water deprivation. The interesting question is why it should persist in doing so when the patient is at risk of drowning in his own juice. The excess fluid is distributed indiscriminately, governed only by hydrodynamic and osmotic considerations. Whereas the primary goal of this compensatory component is to expand circulating blood volume so that the heart can utilize the Frank–Starling mechanism, there is no way for expansion to be restricted in this space considering the nature of the fluid retained; hence expansion of the interstitial fluid space as well (i.e., edema). Because the retained fluid is isosmotic, osmoreceptor stimulation cannot be invoked although it probably continues to play a role in maintaining isosmolarity. General expansion of cardiac chamber volumes in heart failure also precludes volume (low-pressure baroreceptors) receptor mechanism activation.

Since the ADH mechanism does participate in effecting water retention in congestive heart failure, clearly there are other (presumably central) mechanisms for its activation besides osmoreceptors or volume receptors. The renin–angiotensin–aldosterone mechanism also is activated by heart failure. Presumably this is related to relative renal ischemia, especially of cortical nephrons. This becomes a positive feedback system for perpetuating reduced renal blood flow, glomerular filtration, and salt and water excretion, because of the pressor effect of angiotensin II and the salt retaining effect of aldosterone. The possibility exists, therefore, that the salt and water retaining mechanism can overcompensate. This does not seem to be much of a problem in the early phases of heart failure, but it is common in the late stages. It is characterized by fluid retention beyond what is required for optimal cardiac utilization of the Frank–Starling mechanism. The deleterious aspects of such excessive response are that it unnecessarily escalates myocardial tension generating energy requirement without significantly augmenting useful work (lowers myocardial efficiency) and it leads to compromised pulmonary and hepatic function.

It is clinically useful to think in terms of the sidedness of failure; that is, whether primarily of the left or right ventricle. Because systemic capillaries are more sensitive to minor disturbance of the Starling equilibrium, right heart failure produces impressive dropsy that even the patient can detect early in its course. Early pulmonary congestion, however, goes on quietly in the sense that it produces only effort dyspnea (shortness of breath with exercise), something the patient is quick to ascribe to being out of shape or to smoking. Undiagnosed and untreated, it comes on with less and less effort and finally leads to the patient being unable to lie down because of shortness of breath (orthopnea) or to nocturnal attacks that awaken the patient from sleep (paroxysmal nocturnal dyspnea). These manifestations rarely escape the patient's attention and he finally seeks medical attention.

There is a group of heart failure syndromes characterized by absolutely or relatively high cardiac output, so-called high output heart failure. These include thiamine deficiency (beriberi), severe anemia, thyrotoxicosis, chronic severe hypoxemia, and arteriovenous communications. As the term implies, despite typical congestive manifestations, cardiac output at rest is normal or elevated. Clinical reflections of the hyperdynamic circulation include a rapid bounding pulse, active precordial pulsations, and a warm skin.

In thiamine deficiency, high output presumably relates to a defect in oxygen utilization which requires a higher tissue oxygen tension. In thyrotoxicosis, general elevation of tissue metabolic activity (i.e., increased oxygen consumption) requires increased oxygen transport. In anemia and hypoxemia, decreased arterial O_2 content requires a higher blood flow to transport the same amount of O_2 to tissues. Chronic hypoxemia is complicated by the fact that it provokes pulmonary hypertension which tends to reduce output. In arteriovenous communications, output is elevated because of the wasted shunt flow, actual flow to tissues being either normal or diminished. (In this sense, pathophysiology of arteriovenous shunts is more comparable to that in aortic or mitral valve regurgitation and patent ductus arteriosus or ventricular septal defect, disorders in which the left ventricle ejects a larger-than-normal stroke, but only a fraction of it nourishes tissues.)

17
HYPERTENSION

Hypertension, high blood pressure, taken to mean of systemic arterial, is the most common cardiovascular malady that afflicts Americans. Upwards of 20 million—mostly adult—people are estimated to have it. Not only is it common, it is highly significant from the point of view of the severe morbidity and significant mortality associated with it. The only symptom of hypertension per se may be headache, but it exacts its toll by the damage it causes three vital, so-called target organs: the brain, heart, and kidneys. Hypertension causes acute cerebral encephalopathy (cerebral edema), cerebral vascular accidents ("shocks" or "strokes"), left ventricular failure, and acute or chronic renal insufficiency. In addition, there is a strong association between hypertension and coronary heart disease, the leading cause of death in America.

There are many causes of hypertension. Unfortunately known causes account for only a small percentage of all cases, the majority being of the essential or idiopathic (unknown cause) variety. This preponderance becomes overwhelming if systolic hypertension is excluded as a category of secondary hypertension.

Systolic hypertension is the most common form of hypertension associated with a known cause. Its most common cause is a stiff, inelastic aorta associated with atherosclerosis. It is so common with advancing age in civilized societies that it is often considered a normal state of affairs. Undoubtedly it accounts for the gradual increase in the upper limits of normal blood pressure range with age. Other causes of systolic hypertension include aortic valve regurgitation, thyrotoxicosis, and marked bradycardia. Systolic hypertension does not have the hemodynamic significance that diastolic hypertension carries. Except insofar as it is a clue to the presence of atherosclerosis, which has its independent consequences, systolic hypertension usually is tolerated well.

Other causes of so-called secondary hypertension wherein diastolic, as well as systolic, pressure is elevated include: coarctation of the aorta, pheochromocytoma, Cushing's syndrome, primary aldosteronism, unilateral renal artery obstruction, glomerulonephritis, as well as other renal disorders and renal deprivation (renoprival hypertension). When all such causes have been excluded (see the following), it is appropriate to infer that hypertension is primary or essential.

The mechanism of hypertension in the various secondary varieties is reasonably straightforward; that of essential is anything but, although several leads are being pursued including: genetic predisposition, salt intake, psychoemotional response, neuroendocrine factors, absence of vasodilator, and excess of vasopressor substances.

PATHOGENESIS

As pointed out in Chapter 8, the mean blood pressure is determined by only a limited number of variables:

$$\overline{BP} \, \alpha \, SV \cdot HR \cdot \eta \cdot \frac{1}{r^4},$$

where $\overline{BP}$ = mean blood pressure, SV = stroke volue, HR = heart rate, η = viscosity of blood, and r = radius of arterioles.

Obviously there are physiologic limits to the combination of heart rate and stroke volume product that will provide a cardiac output compatible with life at rest (HR minimum 25, maximum 250–300; SV minimum 10 ml, maximum approximately 150 ml). For any given cardiac output and aortic distensibility, mean blood pressure will be the same whatever the HR · SV combination, but systolic and diastolic pressures will vary, the former increasing and the latter decreasing with slow heart rates and vice versa. This is why bradycardia with normal cardiac output produces systolic hypertension even when aortic distensibility is normal.

When a normal stroke volume is ejected at normal frequency into an inelastic (stiff, noncompliant) aorta, systolic pressure is elevated because the windkessel capacitance function is lost. Since potential energy cannot be stored in the rigid walls of major vessels, systolic pressure and flow are increased. This means higher velocity and kinetic energy during systole but less during diastole. Flow in the periphery, therefore, is more pulsatile. Systolic arterial pressure also may be increased (usually modestly) in lesions characterized by large left ventricular stroke volumes being ejected into normally distensible aorta, because the large strokes exceed systolic capacitance and runoff. Diastolic runoff in these conditions is enhanced (aortic valve regurgitation, patent ductus arteriosus shunt or high-peripheral flow in thyrotoxicosis); therefore, diastolic pressure commonly is reduced.

In coarctation of the aorta, the narrowed segment, which usually is just distal to the origin of the left subclavian artery, imposes a resistance in series with that of downstream peripheral arteriolar vascular resistance. How much of a resistance the coarctated segment imposes varies depending on the flow through it. The latter, in turn, depends on the number of collateral vessels and their lumped total conductance and on the flow demands by tissues below the coarctation. For example, at rest, even without collaterals, the narrowing could be as much as a 50% reduction in aortic cross section without being obstructive. During heavy lower extremity exercise, such a narrowing would become significant and lead to the development of some combination of hypertension above the coarctation, hypotension below it, or both. Severe coarctations always lead to development of collaterals, which, because of their tortuosity and long course, are high resistance vessels themselves. Thus hypertension above the coarcted segment is virtually always present.

In all other forms of secondary and in essential hypertension, the fundamental abnormality is the decrease in bore of resistance vessels. There undoubtedly are situations or stages wherein an elevated cardiac output aggravates this underlying defect, but this is not so in the vast majority of cases. The fact that distribution of cardiac output, as well as its absolute level, are normal in the face of variable degrees of hypertension clearly indicates that the vascular obstructive process is generalized. The absence of tissue edema places the locus of obstruction in the arterioles upstream from the capillaries. Thus, these forms of hypertension result from exaggerated arteriolar vasomotion.

One obvious question about hypertension is: What has gone wrong with the barostatic mechanism? Normally, increased pressure in the carotid sinuses and aortic arch causes vagally mediated reflex bradycardia and decreased sympathetic β-, as well as α-adrenoreceptor, stimulation. Their absence has led to hypotheses of a neurogenic basis for hypertension, including inappropriate enhanced sympathetic activity due to baroreceptor resetting (insensitivity), alteration of central mechanisms (vasomotor center, etc.) for blood pressure regulation, increased sympathetic stimulation, or increased sensitivity of vascular smooth muscle to α-receptor stimulation. Evidence for such mechanisms is not consistently found in essential hypertension, but in pheochromocytoma sporadic exaggerated adrenergic stimulation resulting from catecholamine release from an adrenal medullary tumor is the hallmark of the disease. Such patients characteristically have episodic hypertension accompanied by tachycardia and facial flushing. The direct β-adrenergic cardiac chronotropic and inotropic effects and α-adrenergic vasoconstrictor stimulation combine to produce hypertensive crises of troublesome proportions.

The elucidation of the mechanism of Goldblatt experimental renal vascular obstruction hypertension and of clinical hypertension secondary to unilateral renal artery obstruction involving renin release from juxtaglomerular cells of the macula densa, which then acts on renin substrate (angiotensinogen) to produce angiotensin I, which, in turn, is converted to a potent pressor peptide, angiotensin II, by a converting enzyme in the lungs suggested a possible mechanism for hypertension in patients without renal ischemic disease. That is, the renin mechanism might be activated in the absence of overt ischemia or demonstrable obstruction (i.e., increased sensitivity). Its role in essential hypertension continues to be a controversial issue, the complexities of which are only now being investigated.

It was pointed out (Chapter 8) that vasomotor tone was the resultant of all vasoconstrictor and vasodilator influences acting concurrently. The balance point of these varies from organ to organ as evidenced by the insensitivity of cerebral and coronary vessels to α-receptor stimulation whereas those of skin, kidney, and bowel are quite sensitive. Coronary vessels are quite sensitive to hypoxia but not so much so to hypercarbia whereas cerebral vessels are sensitive to both. The distribution of β-adrenergic vasodilator receptors in blood vessels also is variable but there is no doubt that stimulating them causes hypotension. That they are not strikingly tonically active normally is suggested by the minimal primary effect of β blockade on BP. Other powerful vasodilators include vasoactive polypeptides of which bradykinin is the prototype. Prostaglandins of different types have different vascular effects and they are ubiquitous. On the other hand, vasopressin (ADH) is probably the most powerful physiologic pressor substance. This raises the question: Is hypertension the result of an imbalance of one type or another of these substances? Obviously any combination of vasodilator deficiency or vasoconstrictor excess will produce a hypertensive effect. Imbalances of specific vasoactive substances may account for some cases of hypertension, but their role in the vast majority of cases of essential hypertension remains unresolved.

The steady-state salinity of the body varies from individual to individual along with every other physiologic variable. This is because salt intake varies widely as does the ability of the kidney to excrete salt. Since osmolality does not vary quite so much, this means that hydration varies with the salt content of the body. Salt and water retention raise BP, all other things remaining equal. It has been known for some time that salt restriction is often an effective means to lower blood pressure and there is evidence that as a group the hypertensive population consumes more salt on the average than does the nonhypertensive. The effectiveness of thiazide diuretic drugs in reducing blood pressure in a significant percentage of patients with essential hypertension is perhaps the most persuasive evidence of all favoring a role of excess salinity. Hypertension associated with primary hyperaldosteronism, Cushing's syndrome, and deoxycorticosterone administration is based primarily on this sodium retention mechanism. In hyperaldosteronism secondary to hyperreninism, salt retention becomes an aggravating factor. While the role of salt retention in essential hypertension has not been established, it probably is aggravative rather than causal in most cases.

That psychogenic factors may play a role in the pathogenesis of hypertension goes without saying in the context of our society. Just how stress operates to produce vasoconstriction is not entirely clear but an autonomic (sympathetic) component, as least in the early phases, seems almost certain. Epidemiologic data suggest that hypertension is a disorder of civilization. As far as is known, no animals in their natural habitat suffer essential hypertension nor do most members of primitive societies. Small wonder nature has yet to evolve a species-saving mechanism to blunt its effects except in species where hypertension (as defined by human standards) is mandatory such as in the giraffe. The logical conclusion to derive from the foregoing discussion is that while the hemodynamics of hypertension is remarkably simple and the mechanisms of secondary forms reasonably well worked out, essential hypertension is a complex, multifactoral process that, like shock and congestive heart failure, has several possible initiating mechanisms that share a final common pathway that leads to persistent and progressively increasing hypertension that eventually damages target organs.

18
DISEASES OF HEART VALVES

Anatomical lesions of heart valves lead to either or both only two functional defects: obstruction (stenosis) or leakage (regurgitation or insufficiency). There are a number and variety of causes of valve disease including trauma, infection, inflammation, degeneration, tissue redundancy, ischemia (inadequate blood supply) or infarction (tissue death due to loss of blood supply), and stretching of the fibrous valve annulus due to chronically increased tension. Clinical manifestations of valve disorders are related to the specific valve that is involved, which of the two types of defects predominates, the rapidity of progression (or severity of insult, if acute) and the nature of the underlying cause. For example, tricuspid regurgitation by itself is a benign lesion in the presence of normal right ventricular systolic pressure (e.g., posttraumatic tricuspid regurgitation). However, when it is secondary to or associated with severe right ventricular systolic hypertension, manifestations of low cardiac output and systemic congestion are prominent.

The clinical diagnosis of valve lesions is based primarily on auscultatory manifestations. Each valve lesion has a reasonably characteristic constellation of these. Of course, minimal-to-mild lesions may be silent yet easily and unequivocally demonstrable by more senstive specialized techniques. This is particularly true of mitral stenosis and aortic and pulmonic regurgitation because soft murmurs of these lesions are difficult to hear. Very rarely severe mitral stenosis may be found by other criteria in the absence of an audible murmur. Notwithstanding these situations cardiac auscultation remains THE diagnostic screening method for valve disorders and every physician providing primary care should be expert in its conduct.

Auscultatory manifestations, however, are of limited value in quantifying either the severity of valve lesions or their secondary hemodynamic consequences. The clinical history and other physical findings usually are more senstive in such quantification but even they are relatively insensitive. Severe degrees of almost every lesion produce rather stereotyped symptoms and signs that are difficult to miss (although they may be misconstrued) but mild lesions do not.

Before the advent of surgical remedy of valve disorders their precise quantitation was practically academic. While permanent cure of valve diseases has yet to be achieved, surgical and technologic advances have provided remarkable therapeutic benefit, with acceptable operative risk in the vast majority of cases. Thus in most patients it is no longer a case of whether but only when surgical intervention is indicated. The when is determined mainly by the severity of the lesion. This makes it essential to quantify lesions when temporally appropriate by the most sensitive and specific techniques available.

Pure valve (or other cardiovascular) obstructions are easy to quantify hemodynamically if the flow through and the pressure gradient across the obstruction can be measured. These variables permit determination of the degree to which fluid conductance limitation (or resistance increase) has occurred by the simple relationship $G = \dot{Q}/\Delta P$ (or $R = \Delta P/\dot{Q}$) (Chapter 8). In the case of cardiac valves each one transmits the entire cardiac output whereas with other obstructions (e.g., coarctation of aorta, coronary arterial obstruction) some fraction is involved. Flow through valves is intermittent, of course, and the linear Poiseuille relationship for long narrow tubes is not applicable. Therefore, Gorlin and Gorlin modified the short tube formula that permits calculation of orifice cross-sectional area which has proved to be acceptably accurate for clinical purposes. Flow ($\dot{Q}$) is normalized for systolic or diastolic duration as appropriate (depending on whether outflow or inflow valve is involved) and divided by the product of square root of ΔP and an empirical constant which corrects calculated conductance to known orifice dimension

$$\text{Valve area} = \frac{\text{flow/systole or diastole}}{K \sqrt{\Delta P}}.$$

Intracardiac catheterization, a technique demonstrated to be feasible by Dr. Werner Forssman and subsequently to have clinical utility by Drs. Andre Cournand and Dickinson Richards (all received the Nobel Prize), represented a major technological advance for cardiovascular diagnosis. These intrepid pioneers were followed by others such that within a matter of a few decades hardly any intravascular site was beyond the reach of venous or arterial catheterization for the purpose of such flow and pressure measurements, blood sampling or dye (indicator or radiographic) injection.

Angiography, which combines vascular catheterization with sophisticated radiographic technology, permits visualization of cardio-vascular anatomy and function in both static (films) and dynamic (cíne) form. It represents the most useful means for evaluating valve competence, even though it does not provide quantitation of leakage in absolute values with high precision. In atrioventricular valve re-gurgitation gross quantification is possible because the ventriculo-gram can be analyzed graphically to yield total stroke volume from the difference between end diastolic and end systolic ventricular vol-ume. Because forward stroke volume can be measured independently (i.e., cardiac output/heart rate) regurgitation stroke volume is the difference between total and forward stroke volumes. The weakest link in this chain is ventricular volume measurement which involves making assumptions about the geometry of the ventricular cavity.

DYNAMICS OF VALVE OBSTRUCTION

Atrioventricular valve stenosis obstructs ventricular filling whereas that of semilunar valves impedes ventricular emptying. The conse-quences are quite different. Basically obstructive lesions of whatever type or location have the following effects alone or in combination: flow reduction if upstream pressure does not or cannot increase, and increased upstream pressure as the cost of maintaining flow. Clini-cally a pressure gradient develops across obstructions directly pro-portional to the flow rate through and inversely proprotional to the degree of narrowing. Valve stenosis develops insidiously in acquired diseases and when congenital, it develops as cardiac structures de-velop. In the case of semilunar valve obstruction this slow progression allows development of compensatory ventricular hypertrophy (of the so-called concentric type), which distributes increased tension gen-eration requirement among more sarcomeres. This hypertrophy al-lows for higher ventricular systolic pressure according to the Laplace relation, $T \alpha Pr$, while tension developed per sarcomere remains more or less unchanged as long as radius doesn't increase. Thus in semilunar valve obstruction cardiac output is maintained at the cost of ventricular systolic hypertension which increases both external pressure–volume work and internal tension–time heat, as depicted in Figure 18–1. On the other hand, with atrioventricular valve stenosis upstream hypertension is markedly limited because the capacity for atrial hypertrophy as compared with ventricular is far less and up-

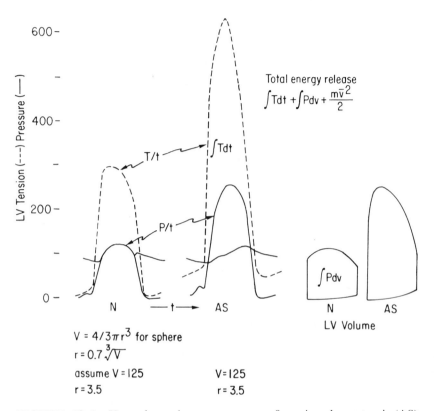

FIGURE 18–1 Hemodynamic consequences of aortic valve stenosis (AS) compared to normal (N). Pressure/time in solid lines and tension/time in dotted lines at left. Pressure volume loops on right. Note pressure gradient during systole between LV and aorta, elevated end diastolic pressure at the same ventricular volume, markedly elevated tension·time ($\int$ Tdt) heat and pressure·volume ($\int$ Pdv) work.

stream hypertension involves the ipsilateral venous compartment as well. Venous hypertension is deleterious because it disturbs upstream capillary fluid dynamics (Chapter 9). On the left side capillary congestion not only is a threat to alveolar respiratory function, it tends to incite secondary pulmonary arteriolar constriction and hypertension. Thus right ventricular outflow obstruction often compounds left ventricular inflow obstruction. It is hardly surprising, therefore, that tricuspid and mitral valve stenosis are accompanied by a combination of flow reduction and upstream pressure elevation. The former is perhaps more prominent with tricuspid and the latter with mitral valve obstructions.

Progressive concentric ventricular hypertrophy associated with semilunar valve stenosis produces diminished ventricular distensibility (or compliance). Greater and greater filling pressure is required to fill the thickened chamber to the same end diastolic volume, as shown in Figure 18–2. This pressure is created by the ipsilateral atrium and the contralateral ventricle. The energy required to fill a ventricle during diastole is dissipated in two forms: pressure–volume and tension–time work. As shown in Figure 18–3, the magnitude of both is small when the ventricle either is distensible or not fully filled. However, they become a significant load, especially for the right ventricle, when left ventricular distensibility is reduced due either to concentric hypertrophy such as in aortic stenosis or to markedly increased ventricular end diastolic volume. Note also in Figure 18–3 that both pressure–volume and tension–time work of ventricular filling are particularly magnified in the terminal phase of diastole when atrial contraction occurs. Diminished ventricular distensibility mag-

FIGURE 18–2 Alterations in ventricular diastolic distensibility associated with various disease processes. So-called concentric hypertrophy (thickening without dilatation) on left of normal associated with left ventricular systolic hypertension. Combined dilatation and hypertrophy curves on right associated with myocardial diseases or those requiring chronically increased left ventricular stroke volumes.

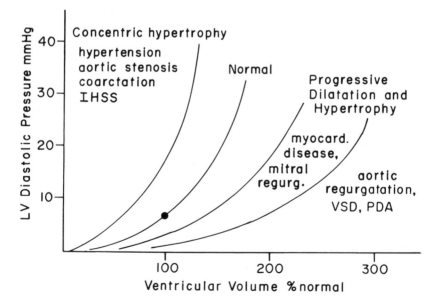

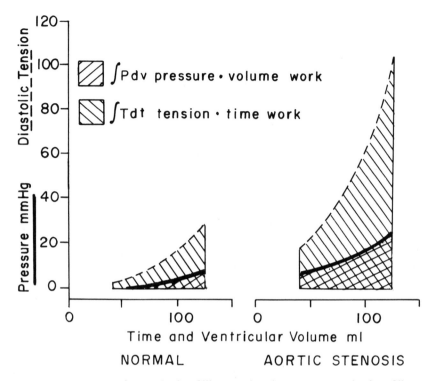

FIGURE 18–3 Left ventricular filling work. The energy required to fill or load the left ventricle is created by the right ventricle and left atrium. The energy is dissipated in two forms stretching the ventricular walls creating wall tension with respect to time ($\int$ Tdt) and filling the chamber along its diastolic volume–pressure curve adding pressure to the blood, that is pressure·volume work ($\int$ Pdv). In the normal heart (left) both components are of a low order of magnitude. However, in concentric hypertrophy such as in aortic stenosis (AS, right) both components increase, especially the tension component because of the Laplace relation.

nifies this effect and explains not only why left atrial hypertrophy is associated with diseases causing concentric ventricular hypertrophy but also the striking deterioration in cardiac performance when appropriately timed atrial contraction is lost in such disorders during various rhythm disorders such as atrial fibrillation, junctional or ventricular tachycardia and A-V conduction blocks. Unfortunately the most common mechanism of atrial fibrillation is left atrial enlargement and hypertrophy. Thus increased filling resistance of the left ventricle on these grounds is an important reason for the old clinical adage: "The most common cause of right heart failure is left heart failure."

DYNAMICS OF VALVE REGURGITATION

In either atrioventricular or semilunar valve regurgitation the added load is encumbered by the ipsilateral ventricle in the form of increased ventricular end diastolic and total stroke volumes. Forward stroke volume is either normal or diminished. As with any hydraulic system, the volume of regurgitation depends on the size of the orifice through which leakage occurs, the pressure gradient between relevant chambers and the time available for retrograde flow. Obviously with atrioventricular valves backward leakage occurs during systole whereas semilunar valve insufficiency is diastolic. Semilunar valves leak due to loss of valve substance (perforation, fibrosis or scarring), leaflet tear or dilatation of the valve annulus. The mechanism of atrioventricular valve incompetence is much more diverse due to the complex valve apparatus. For example, the mitral valve apparatus consists of the left atrium, the mitral valve annulus, the anterior and posterior valve leaflets, the chordae tendineae, the papillary muscles, the left ventricle, and the cardiac rhythm. Anatomic lesions of each of these may cause regurgitation and combinations are common. Rheumatic fever produces mitral valve insufficiency acutely on the basis of valve inflammation and edema and left ventricular dilatation. It subsequently produces chronic progressive regurgitation due to fibrosis and retraction of valve leaflets and chordae tendineae and to annular and left ventricular dilatation. Acute mitral regurgitation associated with myocardial infarction is due to dysfunction of a papillary muscle and the ventricular wall of which it is an integral part (e.g., the wall not only fails to contract it may balloon outward during systole). Bacterial infectious lesions may cause valve leaflet perforation and chordae rupture produces a flail valve leaflet.

Whatever the mechanism and whether of similunar or atrioventricular valve, the hemodynamic consequences of regurgitation depend on the volume of blood regurgitated during each beat for this determines the extra tension–time and pressure–volume work imposed on the ipsilateral ventricle. A normal left ventricle tolerates mild degrees of regurgitation for long duration with impunity. This is accomplished by mild ventricular dilatation and hypertrophy which enables, by means of the length–tension effect, the ventricle to eject the augmented stroke volume without elevation of ventricular filling (and venous) pressure. Regurgitant lesions of a progressive nature or more severe degrees of leakage, especially of the mitral valve, however, tend to culminate in a vicious circle of events wherein the degree of ventricular dilatation is such that tension–time work escalation due to the Laplace effect begets more dilatation and more hypertrophy. At some point ventricular and annular dilatation themselves become a mechanism for mitral regurgitation independent of the inciting mechanism. When the limit of compensatory dilatation–hypertrophy is exceeded, filling pressure begins to rise as the Frank–Starling effect dominates and clinically manifest heart failure results (Figure 18–4).

There are, of course, unfortunate patients who have more than one lesion. These may consist of both stenosis and incompetence of a single valve, stenotic and/or regurgitant lesions of multiple valves, especially mitral and aortic, or combinations of valve disease, hypertension (systemic and/or pulmonary) and coronary ischemic heart disease, each lesion having its contributing as well as compounding deleterious effects. For example, the combination could hardly be worse than that of concurrent mitral regurgitation, essential hypertension and obstructive coronary atherosclerosis. Hypertension compounds mitral regurgitation by increasing the pressure gradient for regurgitation through any given orifice and by aggravating annular and ventricular dilatation because a pressure and flow load are superimposed. Concurrent patchy or global myocardial ischemia limits oxygen delivery to a hypertrophied ventricle whose O_2 demand is markedly enhanced by augmented tension–time and pressure–volume work. The combination of aortic valve stenosis and regurgitation is also exceptionally hemodynamically disadvantageous. The obstruction leads to progressive left ventricular systolic hypertension to provide the pressure gradient during ejection permitting flow to be maintained. Leakage produces effects already discussed: increased diastolic filling for larger stroke volume to compensate for that portion which regurgitates. Enhanced end-diastolic and total stroke volume are the worst possible requirements for a ventricle faced with an outflow obstruction because the combination increases tension–time and pressure–volume work markedly. The discrepancy between left ventricular and aortic root systolic pressures exaggerates extravascular coronary compression coronary blood flow limitation and the

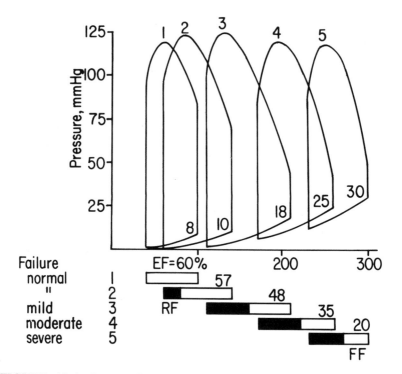

FIGURE 18–4 Stages of progression in mitral regurgitation in terms of pressure volume loops. Normal loop (1) has ejection fraction (EF) of 60%. With mild regurgitation (2) regurgitant fraction (RF) is 25% of total stroke but forward stroke is normal, EF is only slightly diminished and end diastolic pressure is normal. With severe regurgitation (3) total stroke is increased further but RF is now 50% and EF is reduced to 48% because of markedly increased end diastolic volume. Heart failure ensues (4, 5) characterized by diminution in total stroke despite greater edv and edp. EF falls to low levels and RF exceeds forward flow fraction, FF.

diminished aortic diastolic blood pressure associated with leakage represents an insult to diastolic coronary perfusion gradient. It is true that severe degrees of both lesions cannot coexist (i.e., a severely stenotic valve would not permit large volume diastolic regurgitation) but moderate degrees of both certainly can. The markedly increased total energy output requirement (i.e., $\int Tdt + \int Pdv$) associated with such a double lesion is present every beat of the day and night and it is increased still further during periods of exertion. These can be satisfied only by an increase in total coronary blood flow if flow per unit mass of myocardium is to remain undiminished. Because coronary perfusion pressure gradient is fixed (Q = KG), it is obvious that enhanced vascular conductivity (i.e., increased vascularity, vasodilation, or both) may become the limiting factor in compensation for such predicaments. Obstructive coronary atherosclerosis, common in the sex and age group in which aortic stenosis and regurgitation are common, therefore, is a particularly undesirable compounding condition.

NONVALVULAR OBSTRUCTIVE LESIONS

In pediatric practice it is appropriate to consider congenital ventricular outflow obstructive lesions just upstream (infravalvular) or downstream (supravalvular) from semilunar valves. Hemodynamically such lesions produce essentially the same effects as valve obstructions. There is a nonvalvular ventricular outflow obstruction found most commonly in adults that is different. The condition goes by many names, abbreviations of which make a decent alphabet soup: IHSS (idiopathic hypertrophic subaortic stenosis), ASH (asymmetric septal hypertrophy), and SAM (systolic anterior motion of the mitral valve anterior leaflet), to name a few. It is neither a common nor mechanistically uniform condition but it is interesting hemodynamically because it represents a most unusual obstructive lesion that has a dynamic component. That is to say, the presence and/or magnitude of obstruction can vary either from beat to beat or depending on particular circumstances.

Anatomically the outflow channels of the right and left ventricles are different. The right ventricle is more a pass through chamber where blood enters on one side and passes out on a different side. Thus both inflow and outflow channels are completely surrounded by myocardium that comprise the right angled tube. So-called muscular infundibular pulmonic stenosis represents right ventricular outflow obstruction due to hypertrophy of the outflow channel just upstream from the pulmonic valve.

The left ventricle, on the other hand, is a dead-ended, cup-like vessel where the blood enters and leaves on the same side through valves that are side by side. Thus neither orifice channel is completely surrounded by myocardium. Instead, each shares the anterior leaflet of the mitral valve as a limiting boundary during inflow or outflow. During systolic ejection the ventricular aspect of the anterior leaflet of the closed mitral valve forms a portion of the outflow channel. In this situation how could the outflow channel become obstructed below the aortic valve?

The terms IHSS and ASH derive from the idea that the interventricular septum and/or outflow muscular channel hypertrophies out of proportion (asymmetrically) to cause obstruction similar to the mechanism in infundibular pulmonic stenosis. Such hypertrophy can be demonstrated in some patients. In SAM the idea is that instead of moving backward out of the outflow path during systole as it normally does, the anterior mitral valve leaflet moves (anteriorly by echocardiographic direction) into the outflow path to produce obstruction. Such abnormal motion can be demonstrated during ventriculography or by ultrasound (radar) imaging of cardiac structures (echocardiography) in some patients.

The dynamic nature of these mechanisms is illustrated by a number of physiologic and pharmacologic interventions that either precipitate or enhance the obstruction or eradicate or diminish it. These fall into the broad categories of altering either blood pressure or cardiac inotropic state (contractility). Raising blood pressure and reducing contractility tend to diminish obstructions and vice versa.

The clinical consequences of this (these) lesion(s) is in many respects the same as of valvular aortic stenosis. Treatment, however, is less predictable in producing beneficial effects.

Perhaps the important point to be made about valve lesions in a book of this type where physiology is the main concern is that such lesions cause physiologic disturbances whose clinical consequences are reasonably predictable. Early clinical diagnosis of patients with such disorders begins with expert cardiac auscultation for qualitative diagnosis, but competent long-range management depends on understanding how such lesions jeopardize normal circulatory function to produce which clinical signs and symptoms, when which special diagnostic intervention is indicated to quantitate which abnormalities, and when surgical intervention is opportune.

INDEX

Blood flow [cont.]
  laminar, 20
  relationship with velocity, 19, 20
  renal, 170
  skin, 172, 174
  splanchnic, 176–178
  turbulent, 21
  uterine, gravid, 178
  venous O_2 content and, 11
Blood pressure, 96–108, 133–135
  arterial during exercise, 142–145
  arterial in shock, 188
  pulmonary arterial, 153, 155–157
Blood viscosity, 21–23
  anomalous, 22
  effect of red cells, 21–23, 184
  Fahraeus–Lindqvist effect on, 22
  of Newtonian fluid, 22
  of non-Newtonian fluid, 22
  of plasma, 22
Blood volume, 125–131
  and anemia, 187
  antidiuretic hormone and, 128
  and cardiovascular regulation, 130, 131
  determinants, 126, 127
  in hypoxemia, 187
  low pressure mechanoreceptors and,
    129
  osmoreceptors and, 128
  physical conditioning and, 126, 147
  regulation, 127–130
  renin–angiotensin–aldosterone system
    and, 129, 130
Bradycardia, 86, 136
Brain circulation: see Cerebral circulation
Bundle branch, 32
  block, 41, 50

C
Calcium ion
  and contraction mechanics, 61, 62–64
  EC coupling, 57, 58
  plateau potential, 27
Capillaries, 2, 6, 7
  diffusion distance and, 11, 14
  gastrointestinal, 176
  glomerular, 170
  hepatic, 177, 178
  myocardial, 7, 166
  permeability of cerebral, 166
Capillary circulation, 112–117
  dynamics, 113–117
    capillary hydrostatic pressure,
      114–117
    interstitial fluid osmotic pressure,
      116, 117

  plasma osmotic pressure, 113, 114
  Starling hypothesis, 117
  tissue pressure, 116
  in heart failure, 194, 196, 201–203
  pulmonary, 151, 152, 154, 156, 157
  in valve stenosis, 213
Carbon dioxide
  cerebral circulation and, 165
  elimination, 8, 151
  production, 7
Carbon monoxide, 183, 185
Cardiac: see also Heart
  cycle, 67–72, 77
  efficiency, 78, 83
    in heart failure, 196, 197
  energetics, 53, 75–83
    cardiac efficiency, 78, 79
    Frank–Starling law, 75, 76
    pressure–volume loop, 76–78
    tension–time energy, 79, 80
  muscle
    action potential, 26–29
    contractility, 62–64
    contraction, 55, 56
    excitability, 26
    length–tension effect, 31
    plateau potential, 27
    threshold potential, 27
  output, 84–95, 132
    during exercise, 143, 146–149
    in congestive heart failure, 194, 196
    in shock, 188–193
  pump, 53
  rhythm disturbance (arrhythmia),
    47–52
Cardioaccelerator (cardioexcitatory)
    center, 140, 141
Cardioinhibitory center, 134, 140, 141
Cardiovascular reflexes, 132–149
  chemoreceptors, 136, 137
  mechanoreceptors, 133–135
  parasympathetic effector, 132–137
  sympathetic effector, 137–145
Carotid body: see Chemoreceptors
Carotid sinus: see Mechanoreceptors
Cerebral circulation, 164–166
  autoregulation, 165
  blood-brain barrier, 166
  gravity and effect of skull, 164
  vasomotor responses, 165
Chemoreceptors, 136
  cartoid body, 9, 137
  central, 136
Chordae tendineae, 68, 71
Circulation
  function of, 2, 5

Heart [cont.]
  rate
    autonomic control of, 85, 86
    and cardiac output, 89, 91–93, 95,
      132, 134, 135
    in exercise, 87, 91, 94, 146–149
    pacemaker and, 32, 85
  size
    effect of bradycardia, 90
    effect of conditioning, 145
    in species, 88
  sounds
    first, 68, 73
    second, 70, 73
    third, 74
    fourth, 74
    clicks, 74
    opening snap, 74
  valves, 65, 68–72
Hemoglobin
  adult vs. fetal, 17
  effect of 2,3-DPG, 16, 17
  effect of H^+, p_{CO_2}, 17
  O_2 binding, 2, 16
  O_2 saturation, 16, 17
  role in O_2 transport, 15, 16
High cardiac output states, 186, 203, 204
His bundle, 32, 39, 41
Hypertension, 205–209
  essential, 205
  pathogenesis, 206–209
  renin–angiotensin system in, 208
  salt retention in, 209
  secondary, 205
  systolic, 205
Hypertrophy
  cardiac, 163, 199
    in congestive failure, 195
    in overload, 199, 200
  effect on distensibility, 214
  effect on filling work, 215
  skeletal muscle, 55
Hypotension, 130, 131, 188, 189
Hypothalamus
  cardiovascular regulation and, 135, 141, 142
  temperature regulating centers, 175
Hypoxemia
  altitude dependent, 182
  anemia, 183, 184
  carbon monoxide, 183, 185
  fetal, compensation for, 18
  O_2 content in arterial blood in, 15, 183
  polycythemia in, 183, 184
  pulmonary diseases, 183
  veno-arterial shunting, 183

I
Incisura, 70
Inotropy, 62–64, 79–83, 85, 87, 92–95, 140, 148, 168, 169, 195
Internodal tracts, 31, 32
Interstitial fluid, 5, 10, 116, 117, 126
Ischemia, 169, 200
Isometric contraction, 61, 68
Isotonic contraction, 60
Isovolumetric
  contraction, 68
  relaxation, 70

K
Kinetic energy (or work), 76

L
Laplace, law of
  cardiac energetics and, 78, 79
  equation, 23
  right ventricle and, 161–163
  in valve regurgitation, 217
  in valve stenosis, 212
  in work overload, 199, 200
Low-pressure mechanoreceptors, 129
Lymphatic system, 123, 124

M
Mean circulatory filling pressure, 98, 99
Mechanoreceptors, 133–135, 140, 141, 189
Membrane
  muscle
    depolarization, 26, 39
    potassium permeability, 26
    repolarization, 28, 34, 39
    sodium permeability, 26
    threshold, 26
Metabolism, aerobic, 8
Methemoglobin, 185
Mitochondrion
  oxidative phosphorylation in, 8
  O_2 partial pressure of, 8
Mitral valve
  regurgitation, 218
  stenosis, 160, 212, 213
Murmur, 74
Muscle
  electrical properties of, 26
    cardiac, 27–29
    skeletal, 26, 27, 54, 55
  excitation–contraction coupling, role of calcium ion in, 57, 58
  mechanical properties of
    active tension, 59, 60
    force–velocity relation, 61

Respiration
  effect on venous return, 121–122
  tissue, 1
Reynold's number, 21
Rhythm: *see Cardiac rhythm*

S

Sarcolemma, 57
Sarcomere, 55, 56, 60, 63, 64
Sarcoplasmic reticulum, 55–58, 61
Semilunar valves, 68, 69
Shock, 188–193
  blood pressure in, 188
  cardiac output in, 188–193
  definition, 188–193
  heart in, 190, 191
Shunts, 158, 181, 183
Sinoatrial node, 29, 47, 50
  action potential in, 32, 39
Skin circulation, 172–176
  sweat, 173, 174
  temperature regulation, 172–175
sodium ion
  conductance of membrane, 26–28
  in pacemaker potential, 30
Splanchnic circulation, 176–178
  dual hepatic blood flow, 177
  portal hypertension, 177, 178
Staircase: *see Treppe*
Starling hypothesis, 117
Starling's law of the heart: *see Frank–Starling relationship*
Stroke volume, 84, 86–95, 134
Stroke work, 76–78, 82, 197–198, 213, 215
ST segment, 41
Sympathetic nervous system, 85
  α-adrenoreceptors, 139, 140
  β-adrenoreceptors, 139, 140, 159
  cardiovascular regulation and, 137–142
Syncytium, 29, 30
Systole, 65

T

Tachycardia, 48–50, 52, 86
Temperature regulation, 172–175
  core, body, 175
  environmental and skin blood flow, 173
  sweat and, 173, 174
Tension
  in heart failure, 196, 199, 200
  muscle, 30, 31
  -time, 78, 80
  ventricular wall, 78

wall
  relation to pressure, 23
  relation to radius, 23
Tetanus, 55, 57
Thoracic duct, 123, 124
Thyroid hormone, 89
Tight junctions, 30
Transport, circulatory, 7
Transverse (T) tubule, 56, 57
Treppe (staircase), 62
Tricuspid valve
  regurgitation, 210
  stenosis, 201
T wave, 36, 39, 42

U

Umbilical vessels, 179–182
Uterine circulation, 178, 179

V

Vagus nerve, 33:
  see also Parasympathetic nervous system
  atrial myocardium, 85
  atrioventricular node, 33, 51, 85, 189–191
  cartoid sinus massage, 52
  sinoatrial node, 85, 86, 191
  venomotor tone, 191
Valve: *see Heart valves and Venous system*
Varicose veins, 24
Vascular capacity, 127
Vascularity
  capillary density in, 8, 10
  tissue, 8, 9
Vasoconstriction
  α-adrenergic, 139, 145
  heart disease, 143
  mechanoreceptors, 143
  mediators, 138, 144
Vasodilatation
  cardiac output and, 186
  mediators, 139, 144, 145
  in shock, 192
Vasomotor center, 140, 141
Vasomotor tone, 108, 110, 127, 130, 138
  cerebral, 165
  coronary, 167, 168
  pulmonary vascular, 159–161
  in shock, 189, 190, 192, 193
Vasopressin: *see Antidiuretic hormone*
Vasovagal syncope, 136, 145
Vector, 43
  frontal plane, 45
  vectorcardiography, 43
Velocity
  aortic root, blood flow, 66, 67